20-DAY REJUVENATION WEIGHT LOSS PROGRAM

Table of Contents

THE 20-DAY REJUVENATION PROGRAM

PROGRAM BREAKDOWN

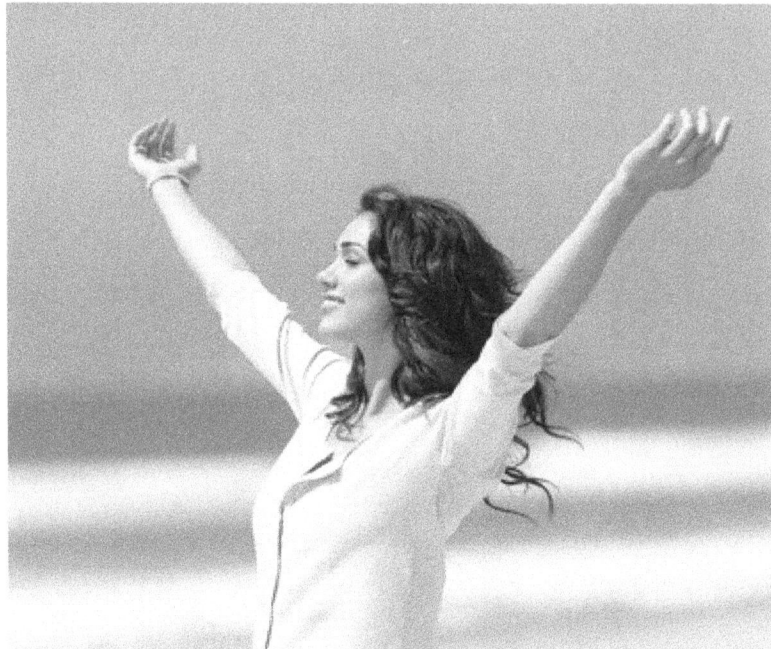

✓	Products and Services Received	Price	Quantity	Total Price
_	20-Day Rejuvenation Supplement Kit	$____.00	_	$____.00
_	Weekly Evaluations	$____.00	_	$____.00
_	Sauna treatments for detoxification	$____.00	_	$____.00
_	Self Mastery Technology (SMT)	$____.00	_	$____.00
_	Follow Up Evaluation	$____.00	_	$____.00
	24 Hours a day phone access to the Doctor and Staff			Priceless!
	Total Price for Everything You Pay			$____.00

The 20 Day Rejuvenation Program

Our goal at Club Reduce is to help the body heal itself naturally. When your body is really healthy, you will arrive at your proper weight.

We want to help educate you on how to live a new and improved lifestyle.

This will not only help you lose the weight you want to lose, but improve every other aspect of your life.

Our doctors have spent over 20 years researching and testing methods with thousands and thousands of patients.

The program you are about to embark upon is a result of all that work.

We seek to provide the most natural ingredients in the highest quality possible, in order to offer the nutrition and building ingredients that the body needs most to reach a level of complete wellness. We follow the preventive health approach, using nutrition and wellness to fight off disease and extra body weight.

We strive to beautify and better the body through researched methods and total programs. These programs are natural, and use the body's own ability to achieve goals of improvement, rather than introducing harmful chemicals, surgery, or addictive drugs.

We want to be a lifetime partner with you in seeking improved health and lifestyle.

We seek constant improvement in our programs, and hope that you will also seek constant improvement in your compliance with a healthy lifestyle.

Our doctors have found that patients who continue to educate themselves on proper nutrition and lifestyle habits achieve great success and maintain that success!

We are honored to partner with you in the new and exciting adventure into improved health!

FOOD LIST

The amount of vegetables consumed on the Herbalogica program is unlimited. Use the list below for successful eating.

- Vegetables may be steamed for four minutes or stir fried over low heat; however, for *best results, ½ of vegetable intake should be raw*.
- Vegetable intake should be twice the amount of fruit intake.
- Use organic whenever possible, frozen is okay, no dried or canned fruits and vegetables.
- Fresh juices made from vegetables and juices are allowed.
- Standard serving size is ½ cup.
- Fresh herbs and spices may be used. Nothing dried.

Vegetables (Always best eaten raw, but if you must cook, lightly steam them)

Artichokes	Eggplant	Pepper, Red
Alfalfa sprouts	Edamame	Pimentos
Asparagus	Fennel	Radish
Bamboo shoots	Garlic	Rhubarb
Bean sprouts	Green Beans	Rutabaga
Beets	Green Onions	Shallots
Bok Choy	Jicama	Snap Beans (Edible Pods)
Broccoli	Kohlrabi	Snow Peas (Sugar Peas)
Brussels sprouts	Lima Beans	String Beans
Buckwheat sprouts	Leek	Sprouts
Cabbage, Chinese	Mung Bean Sprouts	Sunflower Sprouts
Cabbage, Red	Okra	Tomatillos
Carrots	Olives	Tomatoes
Cauliflower	Onion	Turnips
Celery	Parsley	Water Chestnuts
Chard	Parsnips	Wheat Grass
Chives	Peas	Zucchini
Cucumber	Pepper, Green	

Lettuce and Greens

Arugula	Dandelion Greens	Oakleaf
Beet Greens	Endive	Radicchio
Belgian endive	Endigia (Red Endive)	Red Leaf
Bib lettuce	Escarole	Romaine
Boston lettuce	Green Leaf	Spinach
Butter Lettuce	Iceberg	Swiss chard
Cress	Kale	Watercress
Collard Greens	Mesclun	
Curly Endive	Mustard Greens	

Fruits

Apples	Grapefruit	Papaya
Apricots	Grapes	Peaches
Avocadoes	Guava	Pears
Bananas	Honeydew	Persimmon
Blackberries	Kiwi	Pineapple
Blueberries	Lemon	Plums
Boysenberries	Limes	Pomegranate
Cantaloupe	Mango	Raspberries
Cherries	Melons	Strawberries
Coconut (no dried)	Mulberries	Tangelos
Dates	Nectarines	Tangerines
Figs	Oranges	Watermelon

Approved Oils: (Serving size 1 TBSP. if used for dressing, 1tsp for stir fry) use as needed

Coconut Oil – (A great substitute for Butter!)
Extra-virgin olive oil
Flaxseed Oil – (Great for dressings. Keep refrigerated, do not heat)
Grape seed oil
Organic Butter - occasionally
*Use cold-pressed and unprocessed

Salt and Spices:

Salt – Real Salt or Celtic Sea Salt
Any Spices in their whole form. Mixed seasonings generally have sugar or other preservatives.

Juices:

Fresh Vegetable Juices

Water:

Distilled Water (Use during lemonade detox)
Filtered Water
Purified Water
Spring Water
*Remember to drink a minimum of half your body weight in ounces
_____ (body weight)/2=_____ounces of water intake a day

AVOID GROUP:

Alcohol, Caffeine, tobacco or other stimulants
All Coffee and tea (including herbal)
All Dairy – All hard cheese are made from mold. (With the exception of organic butter)
All sugars including: refined sugar, fructose, corn syrup, honey, molasses, date sugar and maple sugar.
(Maple syrup is allowed on detox days)
All white flour and white flour products.
All pastries, bread, crackers, pastas, etc.
Grains

All Meat
Processed or Refined Foods
        Yeast or products containing yeast
        Refined White Flour
        Refined White Sugar
MSG or Chemicals
Starchy Vegetables:
        Hominy
        White Rice
        Yams
        Potatoes
        Corn
        Dried Beans

STRUCTURING YOUR DIET ON THE 20-DAY REJUVENATION PROGRAM

When not detoxing or just juicing, your diet should consist mostly of green leafy vegetables. The easiest way to incorporate more greens into your diet is to plan meals around salads. An easy way to get your daily amount of fruit is to have it for breakfast in the morning or to add it to a Nutritional Shake. Rice and lentils are allowed on the program, but use them sparingly. Add your rice or lentils to a green salad to get more greens in the meal.

Why should my diet consist mostly of raw green leafy vegetables?

Foods that require cooking to be consumed probably are not very good nutritionally for humans. By cooking them, we further compromise their nutritional value, because the vitamins, minerals, enzymes, co-enzymes, carbohydrates, proteins, and fats are damaged or destroyed by the heat of cooking.

Salads are central to a raw diet and should be used to structure your meals. Structure your diet by building every meal around salads. Keep the following tips in mind:

1. Remember that everything you need to live can be found in the produce section.
2. Shop two times a week in order to get fresh produce. Most leafy greens have a refrigerator shelf life of 4-5 days.
3. Buy your produce first. It is the most important food. If you are on a budget, shopping for produce will maximize your dollar as you will avoid junk food while you have a cart full of produce.
4. Wash leafy greens by separating the leaves. Rinse well in order to remove pesticides.
5. Keep your refrigerator well stocked with fresh vegetables. This way you will always have what you need for a salad.
6. While shopping, ask, "How will this go with a salad." Try to consider everything as something that will go into a salad or alongside it.

DETOXIFICATION

The Herbalogica Company is committed to your health, vitality and appearance. We continue to research and develop products and programs that offer total body wellness.

Because of the need for individuals to regularly rid their bodies of accumulated toxins and waste materials, Beneficial International, the parent company of Herbalogica, has spent many years in the development and perfection of the ultimate detoxification and body cleansing program. Designed with the aid and interaction of physicians, nutritionists, and herbalists, the Herbalogica Detoxification Program has helped thousands of people in their quest for health and vitality.

Detoxification is one of the most important factors in the promotion of good health and disease prevention. The Herbalogica Program helps the body to cleanse itself of toxins, mucus and other waste materials in the intestinal tract and major vital organs, improving the way they function. This not only restores new energy to the vital organs, but to the entire body as well.

Herbalogica offers one of the original Detoxification Programs. Our natural formulas have been in use since 1979 – long before detoxification was a popular concept. This history gives you confidence that you are using a program that is safe and effective.

Detoxification can be part of a health maintenance and prevention program when used 3 to 4 times per year. Though it is not a "cure-all", it is a positive way to start addressing many undesirable body conditions, such as allergies, acne, arthritis, skin problems, cellulite, obesity, etc.

Benefits of Detoxification
- An increase in energy is experienced
- The digestive tract can rid itself of accumulated waste and putrefied bacteria. (Typical loss is between 2-8 lbs. of water and waste during a 3 day cleanse.)
- Liver, kidneys and blood are purified and function more effectively.
- The peristaltic action of the colon is strengthened.
- A mental clarity occurs that is not possible under the constant bombardment of chemicals and food additives.
- Physical dependency on habit-forming substances such as refined sugar, caffeine, nicotine, alcohol and drugs is greatly diminished.
- Bad eating habits are broken. As you come off the program, it is easier to make wiser food choices.
- The stomach has a chance to return to normal size, making it easier to control the quantity of food eaten.

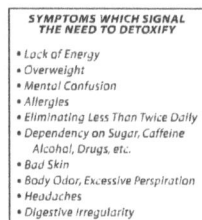

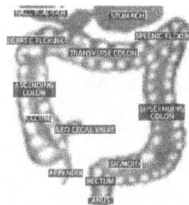

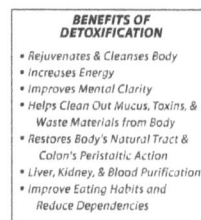

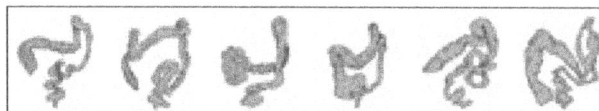

SYMPTOMS WHICH SIGNAL THE NEED TO DETOXIFY
- Lack of Energy
- Overweight
- Mental Confusion
- Allergies
- Eliminating Less Than Twice Daily
- Dependency on Sugar, Caffeine Alcohol, Drugs, etc.
- Bad Skin
- Body Odor, Excessive Perspiration
- Headaches
- Digestive Irregularity

BENEFITS OF DETOXIFICATION
- Rejuvenates & Cleanses Body
- Increases Energy
- Improves Mental Clarity
- Helps Clean Out Mucus, Toxins, & Waste Materials from Body
- Restores Body's Natural Tract & Colon's Peristaltic Action
- Liver, Kidney, & Blood Purification
- Improve Eating Habits and Reduce Dependencies

TYPICAL (UNHEALTHY) COLONS

HEALING CRISIS

The body has natural cleansing abilities that help to expel unnecessary or harmful substances. Four eliminative organs of the body are: the bowels, the skin, the lungs, and the kidneys. These systems are in use all the time, working to keep the body clean and healthy.

When an invader enters the body, the natural process is for the body to remove that invader through eliminative organs. This can happen through diarrhea, vomiting, perspiration (fever), coughing, mucus, or nasal discharge. These natural healing abilities are often under used, as the common response to illness or discomfort is to take chemical medications for symptom relief. We suppress the body's natural eliminative processes through anti-diarrhea drugs, antihistamines, fever reducers, antibiotics and others to keep our bodies from cleansing in the natural way. The "stuffing drugs" that we use drive the virus and bacteria back into the tissues where it can remain until the next immune system crash. Immediate symptoms are managed, but long-term health problems are often the result. For instance, a steroid (cortisone) ointment used for a skin condition may clear up immediate symptoms, but later a more serious problem may occur, such as asthma. In turn, bronchodilators may control the asthma, but may cause depression. In the effort to relieve a patient's symptoms, the real causes of the patient's condition have been overlooked. In addition to environmental toxins and the unhealthy foods that we consume, these types of chemical stuffers contribute to our need to detoxify regularly. A cleansing process such as Detoxification takes these substances out of storage and into circulation to be eliminated. This occasionally causes unpleasant symptoms for a short time. The consumption of caffeine, refined sugar, alcohol and other substances also contributes to the effect that is known as a "healing crisis."

During detoxification and the days following, many people experience some of the signs of a healing crisis, which may include: headaches, skin breakouts, bowl sluggishness, diarrhea, fatigue, sweating, frequent urination, congestion, nasal discharge, or body aches. A few may also briefly experience anxiety, irritability or mental depression.

You must understand that your body is going through cleansing and detoxification. It is throwing out poisons using the energy it has saved from the hard-to-digest meals that have been discontinued. This is your body's natural way of cleansing, and is a positive occurrence.

The best way to encourage your body's natural cleansing methods is to not use over the counter drugs to stop the cleansing process. (Prescription medication should NOT be discontinued without a medical doctor's approval). They may make you feel better in the short term, but to do so by driving toxins back into the tissues. Drink plenty of water facilitate the process and get some rest.

The healing crisis generally lasts from just a few hours to a few days. The healthier one's body is to begin with, the fewer symptoms there will be. The more the body has to clean up, the harder and longer the cleansing side effects will be. Symptoms will also be more pronounced if the change in the diet is abrupt, and less so if it is gradual. This is why detoxification preparation days are so important. Each healing crisis is followed by increased vitality and improved wellbeing.

Please be aware that it is just as important for your body to come off detoxification correctly as it is to detoxify. Your body is in a cleansing mode and will continue until clogging foods are reintroduced. As you finish Detoxification, continue taking the herbs until they are gone. Many of the ill-feeling symptoms that you may have been experiencing will have already begun to disappear. In fact, the three day cleanse is pretty dramatic. You will have lost 2-8 pounds, and will have begun eliminating some of the 5-27 pounds of waste that are being stored in the colon. If you are on medication, ask your prescribing doctor to work with you as you go through this program Start consuming fresh fruit, salads and vegetables. Some people choose to juice live foods for a few days before eating solid foods, allowing the body more time and energy to heal and gain strength. Slowly work your way back into foods after detoxification. Your body is now clean and will no longer tolerate abuse. A couple of beers will make you drunk, and you may become ill after eating pizza, and a candy bar may give you a headache. All these foods are very unhealthy and your clean body is simply more sensitive to toxins.

Contact your Health Care Practitioner for specific questions on Healing Crisis.

Detoxification is a wonderful way to begin a healthy lifestyle. Done 3-4 times per year, the body is cleansed, stronger, and better able to resist illness.

FREQUENTLY ASKED QUESTIONS ABOUT DETOXIFICATION

Will the lemon juice mixture cause too much acid for my sensitive stomach?
Although the lemon is an acidic fruit, it turns alkaline as it is digested and aids in attaining a proper pH balance within the body.

Is detoxification safe?
Absolutely. Body cleansing for health is a concept that has been in use for thousands of years. This type of internal cleanse has been used safely for periods of up to 2 months over the last 30 years. Herbalogica recommends detoxification for 3-10 days only, 3 to 4 times per year. See you Health Care Practitioner for specific directions.

Can I detoxify if I have hypoglycemia?
Detoxifying is especially beneficial to those with hypoglycemia. Just be sure to use only pure maple syrup in the lemon juice mixture. Honey or other sweeteners will trigger an unhealthy insulin response. Herbalogica APPETITE APPEASER will also help to regulate blood sugar levels.

How does detoxification affect cellulite?
Cellulite is waste materials trapped in connective tissue and fat cells, and it is very resistant to ordinary dieting and exercise. While Detoxification will not remove cellulite, it does cleanse the intestinal tract and the body's liquid waste system, thereby speeding up the elimination of toxins from the body, which aids in cellulite removal. Improved results can be achieved when done in conjunction with Herbalogica Body Contouring Wraps.

Will I have energy during the cleanse?

As toxins are expelled from the system, the energy levels rise. It may take a day or two for this effect to occur. If you are not as energetic as you feel you should be, add a little more maple syrup to the lemon juice mixture to raise and maintain your blood sugar level. It is also helpful to make the mixture last throughout the day rather than drinking it all at once. Herbalogica recommends reducing physical activity on detoxification days.

Why is it important to use distilled water?

Distilled water is pure, which means it has no chemicals or bacteria to interfere with the cleansing process. We recommend continuing to use distilled and /or pure spring water after your cleansing program. Do not use bottled mineral water since it may contain concentrations of heavy metals. Soft water is also a poor choice because of its high sodium content.

Will I suffer hunger pains during detoxification?

Yes, you might and if you do, simply drink the lemon juice mixture more often. Since this mixture is food already in liquid form, it gets into the bloodstream faster and allays hunger. You might think you are hungry because you aren't chewing food, but with the mixture you getting the nutrients you need.

Why is it important to use pure maple syrup?

First, pure maple syrup contains many minerals and vitamins. For this reason, it will provide the body with energy. Second, pure maple syrup is a balanced, natural sweetener and can be used without causing an insulin response. Because of this, hypoglycemic's can use the program without fear of lowering or raising blood sugar levels.

Won't the lemon juice mixture cause too much acid for my sensitive stomach? No. Even though lemon is an acid fruit, it turns alkaline as it is digested and aids in attaining a proper pH balance.

SUPPLEMENTS INCLUDED IN THE 20 DAY-REJUVENATION PROGRAM

APPETITE APPEASER
Helps to appease the appetite naturally and lessen nervous tension while dieting. This blend of 11 natural herbs also works together to assist the body in breaking down and dissipating excess fat from around the heart and other vital organs. It also produces the "fat burning" enzymes, and increases energy levels naturally.

BODY PURIFIER
Herbalogica's Body Purifier is a combination of 11 herbs that work together to help rid the liver, kidneys, and bowels of accumulated toxins and other waste materials. Helps to purify the blood stream and cleanse the lymphatic system.

CELLULITE CLEANSE
Stimulates the circulatory system and the lymphatic system to pick up all stored water retention, toxins and waste materials (main contributors to cellulite) harboring in the connective tissues. It then promotes the elimination function for these unwanted substances.

FIBER BLEND
This excellent source of fiber is essential in the fight against obesity. By speeding up the body's food processing time, the important vitamins, minerals, and other nutrients are absorbed from the food. This helps to maximize the body's efficiency without calories. This formula also helps lower cholesterol levels in the blood, cleanses the intestinal tract, and combats constipation.

NUTRITIONAL SHAKE
The Nutritional Shake is an all-natural, 180-calorie, sugar free balanced meal, for healthy weight loss and blood sugar management. This shake easily mixes with water and is available in chocolate, vanilla, strawberry, and orange cream.

INTESTINAL CLEANSER
This formula is a superb combination of 9 herbs that have an extremely beneficial effect on the entire intestinal tract. It is also a bowel tonic and rebuilding formula. It helps improve intestinal absorption of vital nutrients while decreasing the absorption of toxins.

MULTIVITAMIN/MINERAL
Two capsules per day provide 100% RDA of all essential vitamins and minerals. The only way to lose weight permanently, and maintain a well functioning body, is to get 100% nutrition in your diet. Multivitamin/mineral is a great way to get them all into your diet.

VITAMIN D
This easily absorbed liquid gel form of Vitamin D boosts the immune system and helps the body absorb more nutrients. When the body absorbs the proper amount of Vitamin D and the immune system is working smoothly, the risks of disease and infection are significantly lowered. This vitamin also helps with high blood pressure, heart disease, and with depression, which leads to overeating.

How to Take Your Supplements during Your 2-Day Rejuvenation Program

Your Herbalogica supplements are radically different than any other supplements you have taken before. Herbalogica strives to keep their products as pure as possible – unlike a myriad of supplement companies that can allow for a large percentage of fillers in each bottle.

Due to the purity of the product you are receiving, it is essential you follow proper instruction on how to take your daily supplements.

Here are our recommendations:

- Place all your supplements in bags according to the time of day you will be taking them.
    - AM bag
    - PM Bag
- Always take your supplements with food in your stomach.
    - During Lemonade detox days, take with mixture in your stomach.
- Only take 3-4 supplements at a time and wait 30 minutes before taking more.
- Continue this process until all supplements are gone.
- Finish taking all supplements before 6:00pm.

Day 1

Only consume approved fruits and vegetables.

Date:__ /__ /__

AM SUPPLEMENTS:

☐ Appetite Appeaser: 2 | ☐ Cellulite Cleanse: 2 | ☐ Multivitamin/Multimineral: 2 | ☐ Vitamin D: 2

BREAKFAST:	CALORIES	CIRCLE ONE
		Hungry / Emo.
		Hungry / Emo.
		Hungry / Emo.
		Hungry / Emo.
		Hungry / Emo.
		Hungry / Emo.

MIDMORNING SNACK:	CALORIES	CIRCLE ONE
		Hungry / Emo.
		Hungry / Emo.
		Hungry / Emo.

LUNCH:	CALORIES	CIRCLE ONE
		Hungry / Emo
		Hungry / Emo
		Hungry / Emo
		Hungry / Emo

MID-AFTERNOON:		
		Hungry / Emo.
		Hungry / Emo.
		Hungry / Emo

PM SUPPLEMENTS:

☐ Appetite Appeaser: 2 | ☐ Cellulite Cleanse: 2 | ☐ Multivitamin/Multimineral: 2 | ☐ Vitamin D: 1

DINNER:	CALORIES	CIRCLE ONE
		Hungry / Emo
		Hungry / Emo
		Hungry / Emo
		Hungry / Emo

CALORIES YOU ARE ALLOTTED FOR THE DAY:	
TOTAL CALORIES YOU ATE:	

√ = YES x = NO (Check Daily)

- ☐ Follow nutrition guidelines for the day?
- ☐ Did you take all of your supplements today?
- ☐ Did you track your calories?
- ☐ Did you stay within your Calorie Budget?
- ☐ Drink ½ your body weight in ounces? ___oz.
- ☐ Did you exercise? _____ Min

- ☐ Overall, were you hungry when you ate, or did you eat for emotional reasons? (Circle) HUNGRY OR EMOTIONAL
- ☐ If stressed, did you use any relaxation techniques?
- ☐ Write down any questions you have for your next appointment:_____
- ☐ Hours of Sleep received last night _____hrs

Day 2

Date:__ /__ /__

Prep day. Only consume approved fruits and vegetables.

AM SUPPLEMENTS:

☐ Appetite Appeaser: 2   ☐ Cellulite Cleanse: 2   ☐ Multivitamin/Multimineral: 2   ☐ Vitamin D: 2

BREAKFAST	CALORIES	CIRCLE ONE
		Hungry / Emo.
		Hungry / Emo.
		Hungry / Emo
		Hungry / Emo.
		Hungry / Emo.
		Hungry / Emo.
MIDMORNING SNACK:	**CALORIES**	**CIRCLE ONE**
		Hungry / Emo.
		Hungry / Emo
		Hungry / Emo
LUNCH:	**CALORIES**	**CIRCLE ONE**
		Hungry / Emo
		Hungry / Emo
		Hungry / Emo
		Hungry / Emo
MID-AFTERNOON:	**CALORIES**	**CIRCLE ONE**
		Hungry / Emo
		Hungry / Emo
		Hungry / Emo

PM SUPPLEMENTS:

☐ Appetite Appeaser: 2   ☐ Cellulite Cleanse: 2   ☐ Multivitamin/Multimineral: 2   ☐ Vitamin D: 1

DINNER:	CALORIES	CIRCLE ONE
		Hungry / Emo
		Hungry / Emo
		Hungry / Emo
CALORIES YOU ARE ALLOTTED FOR THE DAY:		
TOTAL CALORIES YOU ATE:		

√ = YES x = NO (Check Daily)

☐ Follow nutrition guidelines for the day? ☐ Did you take all of your supplements today? ☐ Did you track your calories? ☐ Did you stay within your Calorie Budget? ☐ Drink ½ your body weight in ounces? ___oz. ☐ Did you exercise? _____ Min	☐ Overall, were you hungry when you ate, or did you eat for emotional reasons? (Circle) HUNGRY OR EMOTIONAL ☐ If stressed, did you use any relaxation techniques? ☐ Write down any questions you have for your next appointment:_____ ☐ Hours of Sleep received last night _____hrs

Day 3 - Detox (Day 1)

Date:__ /__ /__

Notice a change in supplementation and diet today. Today is about cleansing the body!

AM SUPPLEMENTS: Take up to 3 Appetite Appeasers

☐ **Body Purifier: 2** ☐ **Fiber Blend: 8** ☐ **Intestinal Cleanser: 2**

9:00 a.m. – 2:00 p.m.

☐ **Lemon Mixture #1**

☐ **Water Bottle #1**

2:00 p.m.-7:00 p.m.

☐ **Lemon Mixture #1**

☐ **Water Bottle #1**

PM SUPPLEMENTS:

☐ **Body Purifier: 2** ☐ **Fiber Blend: 8** ☐ **Intestinal Cleanser: 2**

√ = YES x = NO (Check Daily)

- ☐ Did you follow the DETOX guidelines?
- ☐ Did you take all of your supplements?
- ☐ Did you drink half of your body weight in ounces? _____oz.
- ☐ Hours of Sleep received last night _____hrs
- ☐ If stressed, did you use any relaxation techniques?

  Rate your stress level today (1=low, 10=high)

  1 2 3 4 5 6 7 8 9 10

Day 4 - Detox (Day 2)

Date:__ /__ /__

Notice a change in supplementation and diet today. Today is about cleansing the body!

AM SUPPLEMENTS: Take up to 3 Appetite Appeasers

☐ Body Purifier: 3   ☐ Fiber Blend: 8   ☐ Intestinal Cleanser: 2

9:00 a.m. – 2:00 p.m.

☐ Lemon Mixture #1

☐ Water Bottle #1

2:00 p.m. – 7:00 p.m.

☐ Lemon Mixture #1

☐ Water Bottle #1

PM SUPPLEMENTS:

☐ Body Purifier: 3   ☐ Fiber Blend: 8   ☐ Intestinal Cleanser: 2

√ = YES x = NO (Check Daily)

- ☐ Did you follow the DETOX guidelines?
- ☐ Did you take all of your supplements?
- ☐ Did you drink half of your body weight in ounces? _____oz.
- ☐ Hours of Sleep received last night _____hrs
- ☐ If stressed, did you use any relaxation techniques?
  Rate your stress level today (1=low, 10=high)

  1 2 3 4 5 6 7 8 9 10

Day 5 - Detox (Day 3)

Date:__ /__ /__

Notice a change in supplementation and diet today. Today is about cleansing the body!

AM SUPPLEMENTS: Take up to 3 Appetite Appeasers

☐ Body Purifier: 4   ☐ Fiber Blend: 8   ☐ Intestinal Cleanser: 2

9:00 a.m. – 2:00 p.m.

☐ Lemon Mixture #1

☐ Water Bottle #1

2:00 p.m.-7:00 p.m.

☐ Lemon Mixture #1

☐ Water Bottle #1

PM SUPPLEMENTS:

☐ Body Purifier: 4   ☐ Fiber Blend: 8   ☐ Intestinal Cleanser: 2

√ = YES x = NO (Check Daily)

- ☐ Did you follow the DETOX guidelines?
- ☐ Did you take all of your supplements?
- ☐ Did you drink half of your body weight in ounces? _____oz.
- ☐ Hours of Sleep received last night _____hrs
- ☐ If stressed, did you use any relaxation techniques?

Rate your stress level today (1=low, 10=high)

1 2 3 4 5 6 7 8 9 10

Day 6 Choose foods from approved food list.   Date:__ /__ /__

AM SUPPLEMENTS:

☐ **Appetite Appeaser: 2**   ☐ **Fiber Blend: 5**   ☐ **Vitamin D: 2**   ☐ **Multivitamin/Multimineral: 2**

☐ **Body Purifier: 2**   ☐ **Intestinal Cleanser: 2**   ☐ **Cellulite Cleanse :2**

BREAKFAST	CALORIES	CIRCLE ONE
		Hungry / Emo.
		Hungry / Emo.
		Hungry / Emo
		Hungry / Emo.
		Hungry / Emo.
		Hungry / Emo.
MIDMORNING SNACK:	CALORIES	CIRCLE ONE
		Hungry / Emo.
		Hungry / Emo
		Hungry / Emo
LUNCH:	CALORIES	CIRCLE ONE
		Hungry / Emo
		Hungry / Emo
		Hungry / Emo
		Hungry / Emo
MID-AFTERNOON:	CALORIES	CIRCLE ONE
		Hungry / Emo
		Hungry / Emo
		Hungry / Emo

PM SUPPLEMENTS:

☐ **Appetite Appeaser: 2**   ☐ **Fiber Blend: 5**   ☐ **Vitamin D: 2**   ☐**Multivitamin/Multimineral: 2**

☐ **Body Purifier: 2**   ☐ **Intestinal Cleanser: 2**   ☐ **Cellulite Cleanse: 2**

DINNER:	CALORIES	CIRCLE ONE
		Hungry / Emo
		Hungry / Emo
		Hungry / Emo

CALORIES YOU ARE ALLOTTED FOR THE DAY:

TOTAL CALORIES YOU ATE:

√ = YES x = NO (Check Daily)

☐ Follow nutrition guidelines for the day?
☐ Did you take all of your supplements today?
☐ Did you track your calories?
☐ Did you stay within your Calorie Budget?
☐ Drink ½ your body weight in ounces? ___oz.
☐ Did you exercise? _____ Min

☐ Overall, were you hungry when you ate, or did you eat for emotional reasons? (Circle) HUNGRY OR EMOTIONAL
☐ If stressed, did you use any relaxation techniques?
☐ Write down any questions you have for your next appointment:_____
☐ Hours of Sleep received last night _____hrs

Day 7 — Choose foods from the approved food list.   Date:__ /__ /__

AM SUPPLEMENTS:

☐ Appetite Appeaser: 2   ☐ Fiber Blend: 5   ☐ Vitamin D: 2   ☐ Multivitamin/Multimineral: 2

☐ Body Purifier: 2   ☐ Intestinal Cleanser: 2   ☐ Cellulite Cleanse :2

BREAKFAST	CALORIES	CIRCLE ONE
		Hungry / Emo.
		Hungry / Emo.
		Hungry / Emo
		Hungry / Emo.
		Hungry / Emo.
		Hungry / Emo.

MIDMORNING SNACK:	CALORIES	CIRCLE ONE
		Hungry / Emo.
		Hungry / Emo
		Hungry / Emo

LUNCH:	CALORIES	CIRCLE ONE
		Hungry / Emo
		Hungry / Emo
		Hungry / Emo
		Hungry / Emo

MID-AFTERNOON:	CALORIES	CIRCLE ONE
		Hungry / Emo
		Hungry / Emo
		Hungry / Emo

PM SUPPLEMENTS:

☐ Appetite Appeaser: 2   ☐ Fiber Blend: 5   ☐ Vitamin D: 2   ☐ Multivitamin/Multimineral: 2

☐ Body Purifier: 2   ☐ Intestinal Cleanser: 2   ☐ Cellulite Cleanse: 2

DINNER:	CALORIES	CIRCLE ONE
		Hungry / Emo
		Hungry / Emo
		Hungry / Emo

CALORIES YOU ARE ALLOTTED FOR THE DAY:

TOTAL CALORIES YOU ATE:

√ = YES x = NO (Check Daily)

☐ Follow nutrition guidelines for the day?
☐ Did you take all of your supplements today?
☐ Did you track your calories?
☐ Did you stay within your Calorie Budget?
☐ Drink ½ your body weight in ounces? ___oz.
☐ Did you exercise? _____ Min

☐ Overall, were you hungry when you ate, or did you eat for emotional reasons? (Circle) HUNGRY OR EMOTIONAL
☐ If stressed, did you use any relaxation techniques?
☐ Write down any questions you have for your next appointment:_____
☐ Hours of Sleep received last night _____hrs

Day 8 Choose foods from the approved food list.   Date:__ /__ /__

AM SUPPLEMENTS:

□ Appetite Appeaser: 2   □ Fiber Blend: 5   □ Vitamin D: 2   □ Multivitamin/Multimineral: 2

□ Body Purifier: 2   □ Intestinal Cleanser: 2   □ Cellulite Cleanse :2

BREAKFAST	CALORIES	CIRCLE ONE
		Hungry / Emo.
		Hungry / Emo.
		Hungry / Emo
		Hungry / Emo.
		Hungry / Emo.
		Hungry / Emo.
MIDMORNING SNACK:	**CALORIES**	**CIRCLE ONE**
		Hungry / Emo.
		Hungry / Emo
		Hungry / Emo
LUNCH:	**CALORIES**	**CIRCLE ONE**
		Hungry / Emo
		Hungry / Emo
		Hungry / Emo
		Hungry / Emo
MID-AFTERNOON:	**CALORIES**	**CIRCLE ONE**
		Hungry / Emo
		Hungry / Emo
		Hungry / Emo

PM SUPPLEMENTS:

□ Appetite Appeaser: 2   □ Fiber Blend: 5   □ Vitamin D: 2   □Multivitamin/Multimineral: 2

□ Body Purifier: 2   □ Intestinal Cleanser: 2   □ Cellulite Cleanse: 2

DINNER:	CALORIES	CIRCLE ONE
		Hungry / Emo
		Hungry / Emo
		Hungry / Emo

CALORIES YOU ARE ALLOTTED FOR THE DAY:
TOTAL CALORIES YOU ATE:

√ = YES x = NO (Check Daily)

□ Follow nutrition guidelines for the day?
□ Did you take all of your supplements today?
□ Did you track your calories?
□ Did you stay within your Calorie Budget?
□ Drink ½ your body weight in ounces? ___oz.
□ Did you exercise? _____ Min

□ Overall, were you hungry when you ate, or did you eat for emotional reasons? (Circle) HUNGRY OR EMOTIONAL
□ If stressed, did you use any relaxation techniques?
□ Write down any questions you have for your next appointment:_____
□ Hours of Sleep received last night _____hrs

Day 9   Choose foods from approved food list.   Date:__/__/__

AM SUPPLEMENTS:

☐ Appetite Appeaser: 2   ☐ Fiber Blend: 5   ☐ Vitamin D: 2   ☐ Multivitamin/Multimineral: 2

☐ Body Purifier: 2   ☐ Intestinal Cleanser: 2   ☐ Cellulite Cleanse :2

BREAKFAST	CALORIES	CIRCLE ONE
		Hungry / Emo.
		Hungry / Emo.
		Hungry / Emo
		Hungry / Emo.
		Hungry / Emo.
		Hungry / Emo.

MIDMORNING SNACK:	CALORIES	CIRCLE ONE
		Hungry / Emo.
		Hungry / Emo
		Hungry / Emo

LUNCH:	CALORIES	CIRCLE ONE
		Hungry / Emo
		Hungry / Emo
		Hungry / Emo
		Hungry / Emo

MID-AFTERNOON:	CALORIES	CIRCLE ONE
		Hungry / Emo
		Hungry / Emo
		Hungry / Emo

PM SUPPLEMENTS:

☐ Appetite Appeaser: 2   ☐ Fiber Blend: 5   ☐ Vitamin D: 2   ☐Multivitamin/Multimineral: 2

☐ Body Purifier: 2   ☐ Intestinal Cleanser: 2   ☐ Cellulite Cleanse: 2

DINNER:	CALORIES	CIRCLE ONE
		Hungry / Emo
		Hungry / Emo
		Hungry / Emo

CALORIES YOU ARE ALLOTTED FOR THE DAY:

TOTAL CALORIES YOU ATE:

√ = YES x = NO (Check Daily)

☐ Follow nutrition guidelines for the day?		☐	Overall, were you hungry when you ate, or did you eat for emotional reasons? (Circle) HUNGRY OR EMOTIONAL
☐ Did you take all of your supplements today?			
☐ Did you track your calories?			
☐ Did you stay within your Calorie Budget?		☐	If stressed, did you use any relaxation techniques?
☐ Drink ½ your body weight in ounces? ___oz.		☐	Write down any questions you have for your next appointment:_____
☐ Did you exercise? _____ Min		☐	Hours of Sleep received last night _____hrs

Day 10   Choose foods from approved food list.   Date:__ /__ /__

AM SUPPLEMENTS:
- □ Appetite Appeaser: 2   □ Fiber Blend: 5   □ Vitamin D: 2   □ Multivitamin/Multimineral: 2
- □ Body Purifier: 2   □ Intestinal Cleanser: 2   □ Cellulite Cleanse :2

BREAKFAST	CALORIES	CIRCLE ONE
		Hungry / Emo.
		Hungry / Emo.
		Hungry / Emo
		Hungry / Emo.
		Hungry / Emo.
		Hungry / Emo.
MIDMORNING SNACK:	**CALORIES**	**CIRCLE ONE**
		Hungry / Emo.
		Hungry / Emo
		Hungry / Emo
LUNCH:	**CALORIES**	**CIRCLE ONE**
		Hungry / Emo
		Hungry / Emo
		Hungry / Emo
		Hungry / Emo
MID-AFTERNOON:	**CALORIES**	**CIRCLE ONE**
		Hungry / Emo
		Hungry / Emo
		Hungry / Emo

PM SUPPLEMENTS:
- □ Appetite Appeaser: 2   □ Fiber Blend: 5   □ Vitamin D: 2   □ Multivitamin/Multimineral: 2
- □ Body Purifier: 2   □ Intestinal Cleanser: 2   □ Cellulite Cleanse: 2

DINNER:	CALORIES	CIRCLE ONE
		Hungry / Emo
		Hungry / Emo
		Hungry / Emo

CALORIES YOU ARE ALLOTTED FOR THE DAY:

TOTAL CALORIES YOU ATE:

√ = YES x = NO (Check Daily)

□ Follow nutrition guidelines for the day?	□ Overall, were you hungry when you ate, or did you eat for emotional reasons? (Circle) HUNGRY OR EMOTIONAL
□ Did you take all of your supplements today?	
□ Did you track your calories?	
□ Did you stay within your Calorie Budget?	□ If stressed, did you use any relaxation techniques?
□ Drink ½ your body weight in ounces? ___oz.	
□ Did you exercise? _____ Min	□ Write down any questions you have for your next appointment:_____
	□ Hours of Sleep received last night _____hrs

Day 11 Choose foods from the approved list. Date:__ /__ /__

AM SUPPLEMENTS:
☐ Appetite Appeaser: 2   ☐ Fiber Blend: 5   ☐ Vitamin D: 2   ☐ Multivitamin/Multimineral: 2
☐ Body Purifier: 2   ☐ Intestinal Cleanser: 2   ☐ Cellulite Cleanse :2

BREAKFAST	CALORIES	CIRCLE ONE
		Hungry / Emo.
		Hungry / Emo.
		Hungry / Emo
		Hungry / Emo.
		Hungry / Emo.
		Hungry / Emo.
MIDMORNING SNACK:	CALORIES	CIRCLE ONE
		Hungry / Emo.
		Hungry / Emo
		Hungry / Emo
LUNCH:	CALORIES	CIRCLE ONE
		Hungry / Emo
		Hungry / Emo
		Hungry / Emo
		Hungry / Emo
MID-AFTERNOON:	CALORIES	CIRCLE ONE
		Hungry / Emo
		Hungry / Emo
		Hungry / Emo

PM SUPPLEMENTS:
☐ Appetite Appeaser: 2   ☐ Fiber Blend: 5   ☐ Vitamin D: 2   ☐ Multivitamin/Multimineral: 2
☐ Body Purifier: 2   ☐ Intestinal Cleanser: 2   ☐ Cellulite Cleanse: 2

DINNER:	CALORIES	CIRCLE ONE
		Hungry / Emo
		Hungry / Emo
		Hungry / Emo

CALORIES YOU ARE ALLOTTED FOR THE DAY:
TOTAL CALORIES YOU ATE:

√ = YES x = NO (Check Daily)

☐ Follow nutrition guidelines for the day?
☐ Did you take all of your supplements today?
☐ Did you track your calories?
☐ Did you stay within your Calorie Budget?
☐ Drink ½ your body weight in ounces? ___oz.
☐ Did you exercise? _____ Min

☐ Overall, were you hungry when you ate, or did you eat for emotional reasons? (Circle) HUNGRY OR EMOTIONAL
☐ If stressed, did you use any relaxation techniques?
☐ Write down any questions you have for your next appointment:_____
☐ Hours of Sleep received last night _____hrs

Day 12 Choose foods from the approved list.   Date:__ /__ /__

AM SUPPLEMENTS:
- Appetite Appeaser: 2
- Body Purifier: 2
- Fiber Blend: 5
- Intestinal Cleanser: 2
- Vitamin D: 2
- Cellulite Cleanse :2
- Multivitamin/Multimineral: 2

BREAKFAST	CALORIES	CIRCLE ONE
		Hungry / Emo.
		Hungry / Emo.
		Hungry / Emo
		Hungry / Emo.
		Hungry / Emo.
		Hungry / Emo.
MIDMORNING SNACK:	CALORIES	CIRCLE ONE
		Hungry / Emo.
		Hungry / Emo
		Hungry / Emo
LUNCH:	CALORIES	CIRCLE ONE
		Hungry / Emo
		Hungry / Emo
		Hungry / Emo
		Hungry / Emo
MID-AFTERNOON:	CALORIES	CIRCLE ONE
		Hungry / Emo
		Hungry / Emo
		Hungry / Emo

PM SUPPLEMENTS:
- Appetite Appeaser: 2
- Body Purifier: 2
- Fiber Blend: 5
- Intestinal Cleanser: 2
- Vitamin D: 2
- Cellulite Cleanse: 2
- Multivitamin/Multimineral: 2

DINNER:	CALORIES	CIRCLE ONE
		Hungry / Emo
		Hungry / Emo
		Hungry / Emo

CALORIES YOU ARE ALLOTTED FOR THE DAY:
TOTAL CALORIES YOU ATE:

√ = YES x = NO (Check Daily)

- ☐ Follow nutrition guidelines for the day?
- ☐ Did you take all of your supplements today?
- ☐ Did you track your calories?
- ☐ Did you stay within your Calorie Budget?
- ☐ Drink ½ your body weight in ounces? ___oz.
- ☐ Did you exercise? _____ Min

- ☐ Overall, were you hungry when you ate, or did you eat for emotional reasons? (Circle) HUNGRY OR EMOTIONAL
- ☐ If stressed, did you use any relaxation techniques?
- ☐ Write down any questions you have for your next appointment:_____
- ☐ Hours of Sleep received last night _____hrs

Day 13 Choose food from the approved list.   Date:__ /__ /__

AM SUPPLEMENTS:

□ Appetite Appeaser: 2   □ Fiber Blend: 5   □ Vitamin D: 2   □ Multivitamin/Multimineral: 2

□ Body Purifier: 2   □ Intestinal Cleanser: 2   □ Cellulite Cleanse :2

BREAKFAST	CALORIES	CIRCLE ONE
		Hungry / Emo.
		Hungry / Emo.
		Hungry / Emo
		Hungry / Emo.
		Hungry / Emo.
		Hungry / Emo.

MIDMORNING SNACK:	CALORIES	CIRCLE ONE
		Hungry / Emo.
		Hungry / Emo
		Hungry / Emo

LUNCH:	CALORIES	CIRCLE ONE
		Hungry / Emo
		Hungry / Emo
		Hungry / Emo
		Hungry / Emo

MID-AFTERNOON:	CALORIES	CIRCLE ONE
		Hungry / Emo
		Hungry / Emo
		Hungry / Emo

PM SUPPLEMENTS:

□ Appetite Appeaser: 2   □ Fiber Blend: 5   □ Vitamin D: 2   □Multivitamin/Multimineral: 2

□ Body Purifier: 2   □ Intestinal Cleanser: 2   □ Cellulite Cleanse: 2

DINNER:	CALORIES	CIRCLE ONE
		Hungry / Emo
		Hungry / Emo
		Hungry / Emo

CALORIES YOU ARE ALLOTTED FOR THE DAY:

TOTAL CALORIES YOU ATE:

√ = YES x = NO (Check Daily)

□ Follow nutrition guidelines for the day? □ Did you take all of your supplements today? □ Did you track your calories? □ Did you stay within your Calorie Budget? □ Drink ½ your body weight in ounces? ___oz. □ Did you exercise? _____ Min	□ Overall, were you hungry when you ate, or did you eat for emotional reasons? (Circle) HUNGRY OR EMOTIONAL □ If stressed, did you use any relaxation techniques? □ Write down any questions you have for your next appointment:_____ □ Hours of Sleep received last night _____hrs

Day 14 Choose food from the approved list.   Date:__ /__ /__

AM SUPPLEMENTS:

☐ Appetite Appeaser: 2   ☐ Fiber Blend: 5   ☐ Vitamin D: 2   ☐ Multivitamin/Multimineral: 2
☐ Body Purifier: 2   ☐ Intestinal Cleanser: 2   ☐ Cellulite Cleanse :2

BREAKFAST	CALORIES	CIRCLE ONE
		Hungry / Emo.
		Hungry / Emo.
		Hungry / Emo
		Hungry / Emo.
		Hungry / Emo.
		Hungry / Emo.
MIDMORNING SNACK:	**CALORIES**	**CIRCLE ONE**
		Hungry / Emo.
		Hungry / Emo
		Hungry / Emo
LUNCH:	**CALORIES**	**CIRCLE ONE**
		Hungry / Emo
		Hungry / Emo
		Hungry / Emo
		Hungry / Emo
MID-AFTERNOON:	**CALORIES**	**CIRCLE ONE**
		Hungry / Emo
		Hungry / Emo
		Hungry / Emo

PM SUPPLEMENTS:

☐ Appetite Appeaser: 2   ☐ Fiber Blend: 5   ☐ Vitamin D: 2   ☐ Multivitamin/Multimineral: 2
☐ Body Purifier: 2   ☐ Intestinal Cleanser: 2   ☐ Cellulite Cleanse: 2

DINNER:	CALORIES	CIRCLE ONE
		Hungry / Emo
		Hungry / Emo
		Hungry / Emo

CALORIES YOU ARE ALLOTTED FOR THE DAY:
TOTAL CALORIES YOU ATE:

√ = YES x = NO (Check Daily)

☐ Follow nutrition guidelines for the day?
☐ Did you take all of your supplements today?
☐ Did you track your calories?
☐ Did you stay within your Calorie Budget?
☐ Drink ½ your body weight in ounces? ___oz.
☐ Did you exercise? _____ Min

☐ Overall, were you hungry when you ate, or did you eat for emotional reasons? (Circle) HUNGRY OR EMOTIONAL
☐ If stressed, did you use any relaxation techniques?
☐ Write down any questions you have for your next appointment:_____
☐ Hours of Sleep received last night _____hrs

Day 15   Choose foods from the approved list.   Date:__ /__ /__

AM SUPPLEMENTS:

☐ Appetite Appeaser: 2   ☐ Fiber Blend: 5   ☐ Vitamin D: 2   ☐ Multivitamin/Multimineral: 2
☐ Body Purifier: 2   ☐ Intestinal Cleanser: 2   ☐ Cellulite Cleanse :2

BREAKFAST	CALORIES	CIRCLE ONE
		Hungry / Emo.
		Hungry / Emo.
		Hungry / Emo
		Hungry / Emo.
		Hungry / Emo.
		Hungry / Emo.

MIDMORNING SNACK:	CALORIES	CIRCLE ONE
		Hungry / Emo.
		Hungry / Emo
		Hungry / Emo

LUNCH:	CALORIES	CIRCLE ONE
		Hungry / Emo
		Hungry / Emo
		Hungry / Emo
		Hungry / Emo

MID-AFTERNOON:	CALORIES	CIRCLE ONE
		Hungry / Emo
		Hungry / Emo
		Hungry / Emo

PM SUPPLEMENTS:

☐ Appetite Appeaser: 2   ☐ Fiber Blend: 5   ☐ Vitamin D: 2   ☐Multivitamin/Multimineral: 2
☐ Body Purifier: 2   ☐ Intestinal Cleanser: 2   ☐ Cellulite Cleanse: 2

DINNER:	CALORIES	CIRCLE ONE
		Hungry / Emo
		Hungry / Emo
		Hungry / Emo

CALORIES YOU ARE ALLOTTED FOR THE DAY:

TOTAL CALORIES YOU ATE:

√ = YES x = NO (Check Daily)

☐ Follow nutrition guidelines for the day?	☐ Overall, were you hungry when you ate, or did you eat for emotional reasons? (Circle) HUNGRY OR EMOTIONAL
☐ Did you take all of your supplements today?	
☐ Did you track your calories?	
☐ Did you stay within your Calorie Budget?	☐ If stressed, did you use any relaxation techniques?
☐ Drink ½ your body weight in ounces? ___oz.	☐ Write down any questions you have for your next appointment:_____
☐ Did you exercise? _____ Min	☐ Hours of Sleep received last night _____hrs

Day 16   Choose foods from the approved list.   Date:__ /__ /__

AM SUPPLEMENTS:
- ☐ Appetite Appeaser: 2   ☐ Fiber Blend: 5   ☐ Vitamin D: 2   ☐ Multivitamin/ Multimineral: 2
- ☐ Body Purifier: 2   ☐ Intestinal Cleanser: 2   ☐ Cellulite Cleanse :2

BREAKFAST	CALORIES	CIRCLE ONE
		Hungry / Emo.
		Hungry / Emo.
		Hungry / Emo
		Hungry / Emo.
		Hungry / Emo.
		Hungry / Emo.
MIDMORNING SNACK:	**CALORIES**	**CIRCLE ONE**
		Hungry / Emo.
		Hungry / Emo
		Hungry / Emo
LUNCH:	**CALORIES**	**CIRCLE ONE**
		Hungry / Emo
		Hungry / Emo
		Hungry / Emo
		Hungry / Emo
MID-AFTERNOON:	**CALORIES**	**CIRCLE ONE**
		Hungry / Emo
		Hungry / Emo
		Hungry / Emo

PM SUPPLEMENTS:
- ☐ Appetite Appeaser: 2   ☐ Fiber Blend: 5   ☐ Vitamin D: 2   ☐ Multivitamin/Multimineral: 2
- ☐ Body Purifier: 2   ☐ Intestinal Cleanser: 2   ☐ Cellulite Cleanse: 2

DINNER:	CALORIES	CIRCLE ONE
		Hungry / Emo
		Hungry / Emo
		Hungry / Emo

CALORIES YOU ARE ALLOTTED FOR THE DAY:

TOTAL CALORIES YOU ATE:

√ = YES x = NO (Check Daily)

☐ Follow nutrition guidelines for the day? ☐ Did you take all of your supplements today? ☐ Did you track your calories? ☐ Did you stay within your Calorie Budget? ☐ Drink ½ your body weight in ounces? ___oz. ☐ Did you exercise? _____ Min	☐ Overall, were you hungry when you ate, or did you eat for emotional reasons? (Circle) HUNGRY OR EMOTIONAL ☐ If stressed, did you use any relaxation techniques? ☐ Write down any questions you have for your next appointment:_____ ☐ Hours of Sleep received last night _____hrs

Day 17 Choose foods from the approved list.   Date:__ /__ /__

AM SUPPLEMENTS:
☐ Appetite Appeaser: 2   ☐ Fiber Blend: 5   ☐ Vitamin D: 2   ☐ Multivitamin/ Multimineral: 2
☐ Body Purifier: 2   ☐ Intestinal Cleanser: 2   ☐ Cellulite Cleanse :2

BREAKFAST	CALORIES	CIRCLE ONE
		Hungry / Emo.
		Hungry / Emo.
		Hungry / Emo
		Hungry / Emo.
		Hungry / Emo.
		Hungry / Emo.
MIDMORNING SNACK:	**CALORIES**	**CIRCLE ONE**
		Hungry / Emo.
		Hungry / Emo
		Hungry / Emo
LUNCH:	**CALORIES**	**CIRCLE ONE**
		Hungry / Emo
		Hungry / Emo
		Hungry / Emo
		Hungry / Emo
MID-AFTERNOON:	**CALORIES**	**CIRCLE ONE**
		Hungry / Emo
		Hungry / Emo
		Hungry / Emo

PM SUPPLEMENTS:
☐ Appetite Appeaser: 2   ☐ Fiber Blend: 5   ☐ Vitamin D: 2   ☐ Multivitamin/Multimineral: 2
☐ Body Purifier: 2   ☐ Intestinal Cleanser: 2   ☐ Cellulite Cleanse: 2

DINNER:	CALORIES	CIRCLE ONE
		Hungry / Emo
		Hungry / Emo
		Hungry / Emo

CALORIES YOU ARE ALLOTTED FOR THE DAY:

TOTAL CALORIES YOU ATE:

√ = YES x = NO (Check Daily)

☐ Follow nutrition guidelines for the day?	☐ Overall, were you hungry when you ate, or did you eat for emotional reasons? (Circle) HUNGRY OR EMOTIONAL
☐ Did you take all of your supplements today?	
☐ Did you track your calories?	
☐ Did you stay within your Calorie Budget?	☐ If stressed, did you use any relaxation techniques?
☐ Drink ½ your body weight in ounces? ___oz.	☐ Write down any questions you have for your next appointment:_____
☐ Did you exercise? _____ Min	☐ Hours of Sleep received last night _____hrs

Day 18 Choose foods from the approved list.

Date:__ /__ /__

AM SUPPLEMENTS:

☐ Appetite Appeaser: 2 ☐ Fiber Blend: 5 ☐ Vitamin D: 2 ☐ Multivitamin/ Multimineral: 2

☐ Body Purifier: 2 ☐ Intestinal Cleanser: 2 ☐ Cellulite Cleanse :2

BREAKFAST	CALORIES	CIRCLE ONE
		Hungry / Emo.
		Hungry / Emo.
		Hungry / Emo
		Hungry / Emo.
		Hungry / Emo.
		Hungry / Emo.
MIDMORNING SNACK:	**CALORIES**	**CIRCLE ONE**
		Hungry / Emo.
		Hungry / Emo
		Hungry / Emo
LUNCH:	**CALORIES**	**CIRCLE ONE**
		Hungry / Emo
		Hungry / Emo
		Hungry / Emo
		Hungry / Emo
MID-AFTERNOON:	**CALORIES**	**CIRCLE ONE**
		Hungry / Emo
		Hungry / Emo
		Hungry / Emo

PM SUPPLEMENTS:

☐ Appetite Appeaser: 2 ☐ Fiber Blend: 5 ☐ Vitamin D: 2 ☐ Multivitamin/Multimineral: 2

☐ Body Purifier: 2 ☐ Intestinal Cleanser: 2 ☐ Cellulite Cleanse: 2

DINNER:	CALORIES	CIRCLE ONE
		Hungry / Emo
		Hungry / Emo
		Hungry / Emo

CALORIES YOU ARE ALLOTTED FOR THE DAY:

TOTAL CALORIES YOU ATE:

√ = YES x = NO (Check Daily)

☐ Follow nutrition guidelines for the day? ☐ Did you take all of your supplements today? ☐ Did you track your calories? ☐ Did you stay within your Calorie Budget? ☐ Drink ½ your body weight in ounces? ___oz. ☐ Did you exercise? _____ Min	☐ Overall, were you hungry when you ate, or did you eat for emotional reasons? (Circle) HUNGRY OR EMOTIONAL ☐ If stressed, did you use any relaxation techniques? ☐ Write down any questions you have for your next appointment:_____ ☐ Hours of Sleep received last night _____hrs

Day 19 Choose foods from the approved food list.   Date:__ /__ /__

AM SUPPLEMENTS:
☐ Appetite Appeaser: 2   ☐ Fiber Blend: 5   ☐ Vitamin D: 2   ☐ Multivitamin/ Multimineral: 2
☐ Body Purifier: 2   ☐ Intestinal Cleanser: 2   ☐ Cellulite Cleanse :2

BREAKFAST	CALORIES	CIRCLE ONE
		Hungry / Emo.
		Hungry / Emo.
		Hungry / Emo
		Hungry / Emo.
		Hungry / Emo.
		Hungry / Emo.
MIDMORNING SNACK:	**CALORIES**	**CIRCLE ONE**
		Hungry / Emo.
		Hungry / Emo
		Hungry / Emo
LUNCH:	**CALORIES**	**CIRCLE ONE**
		Hungry / Emo
		Hungry / Emo
		Hungry / Emo
		Hungry / Emo
MID-AFTERNOON:	**CALORIES**	**CIRCLE ONE**
		Hungry / Emo
		Hungry / Emo
		Hungry / Emo

PM SUPPLEMENTS:
☐ Appetite Appeaser: 2   ☐ Fiber Blend: 5   ☐ Vitamin D: 2   ☐ Multivitamin/Multimineral: 2
☐ Body Purifier: 2   ☐ Intestinal Cleanser: 2   ☐ Cellulite Cleanse: 2

DINNER:	CALORIES	CIRCLE ONE
		Hungry / Emo
		Hungry / Emo
		Hungry / Emo

CALORIES YOU ARE ALLOTTED FOR THE DAY:

TOTAL CALORIES YOU ATE:

√ = YES x = NO (Check Daily)

☐ Follow nutrition guidelines for the day?	☐ Overall, were you hungry when you ate, or did you eat for emotional reasons? (Circle) HUNGRY OR EMOTIONAL
☐ Did you take all of your supplements today?	
☐ Did you track your calories?	☐ If stressed, did you use any relaxation techniques?
☐ Did you stay within your Calorie Budget?	
☐ Drink ½ your body weight in ounces? ___oz.	☐ Write down any questions you have for your next appointment:_____
☐ Did you exercise? _____ Min	☐ Hours of Sleep received last night _____hrs

Day 20 Choose foods from the approved list.   Date:__ /__ /__

AM SUPPLEMENTS:
☐ Appetite Appeaser: 2   ☐ Fiber Blend: 5   ☐ Vitamin D: 2   ☐ Multivitamin/Multimineral: 2
☐ Body Purifier: 2   ☐ Intestinal Cleanser: 2   ☐ Cellulite Cleanse :2

BREAKFAST	CALORIES	CIRCLE ONE
		Hungry / Emo.
		Hungry / Emo.
		Hungry / Emo
		Hungry / Emo.
		Hungry / Emo.
		Hungry / Emo.
MIDMORNING SNACK:	**CALORIES**	**CIRCLE ONE**
		Hungry / Emo.
		Hungry / Emo
		Hungry / Emo
LUNCH:	**CALORIES**	**CIRCLE ONE**
		Hungry / Emo
		Hungry / Emo
		Hungry / Emo
		Hungry / Emo
MID-AFTERNOON:	**CALORIES**	**CIRCLE ONE**
		Hungry / Emo
		Hungry / Emo
		Hungry / Emo

PM SUPPLEMENTS:
☐ Appetite Appeaser: 2   ☐ Fiber Blend: 5   ☐ Vitamin D: 2   ☐ Multivitamin/Multimineral: 2
☐ Body Purifier: 2   ☐ Intestinal Cleanser: 2   ☐ Cellulite Cleanse: 2

DINNER:	CALORIES	CIRCLE ONE
		Hungry / Emo
		Hungry / Emo
		Hungry / Emo

CALORIES YOU ARE ALLOTTED FOR THE DAY:

TOTAL CALORIES YOU ATE:

√ = YES x = NO (Check Daily)

☐ Follow nutrition guidelines for the day? ☐ Did you take all of your supplements today? ☐ Did you track your calories? ☐ Did you stay within your Calorie Budget? ☐ Drink ½ your body weight in ounces? ___oz. ☐ Did you exercise? _____ Min	☐ Overall, were you hungry when you ate, or did you eat for emotional reasons? (Circle) HUNGRY OR EMOTIONAL ☐ If stressed, did you use any relaxation techniques? ☐ Write down any questions you have for your next appointment:_____ ☐ Hours of Sleep received last night _____hrs

DAY 21 and Beyond

Once someone has gone through a 20 DAY REJUVENATION Program, they should be feeling like a completely new person. A new level of vitality and health will have been reached. Now each person must decide how they will live to maintain this level of wellness, and even improve upon it. Use the following list to ensure lasting health:

- Body cleansing and detoxification — everyone should detoxify at least four times per year. We still live in a toxic society, and this becomes a cleansing lifestyle.
- Proper food choices — consist of foods that heal the body, rather than foods that destroy health.
- Exercise — at least 40 minutes per day. Alternate weight-bearing and cardiovascular.
- Learn to deal positively with stress.
- Listen to the body. The body will tell you what it needs and what it doesn't need.
- Become educated on how the body works.
- Live a positive, happy, healthy life.
- 100% nutrition — there will always be a need to supplement nutrients, as it is impossible to get complete nutrition by eating food sources as they are in today's world.
- Herbalogica recommends these supplements each day for a healthy body
    - Multivitamin / Multimineral
    - Antioxidant
    - Flax Seed Oil
    - Evening Primrose Oil
    - Vitamin D
    - Liquid Calcium
    - Digestive Enzyme
    - Herbalogica Nutritional Shake
- Eat twice as many veggies as fruits
- Eat a variety of foods and a rainbow of colors
- Fresh and organic produce is always best
- Have one Herbalogica Nutritional shake daily to replace a meal
- Take all recommended supplements – ask about specific supplementation for your particular needs
- If using salt, use Real Salt or Sea Salt
- DRINK WATER: You should be drinking half your weight in ounces – not tap water!
- Get to bed early and get 8 hours of sleep if possible
- No processed foods!
- No MSG and NO CHEMICALS
- 5-7 small meals throughout the day will keep your metabolism going
- Last meal of the day should be eaten before 6 pm
- Track calories, Women: 1000-1100 calories per day, Men: 1200-1300 calories per day

RECIPES

Shakes

Chocolate Dream		5 mins	Serves 1
<ul><li>2 scoops Herbalogica Chocolate</li><li>1 cup ice cubes</li></ul>	<ul><li>1 cup water</li></ul>		
Combine all ingredients in a blender and blend well.			
✓ LOVED IT!	✓ Didn't like it		

Fruit Smoothie	5 mins	Serves 1
<ul><li>2 oranges</li><li>1 banana</li><li>½ cup berries</li><li>2 scoops Herbalogica Vanilla</li></ul>		
Combine all ingredients in a blender and blend well.		
✓ LOVED IT! ✓ Didn't like it		

Pina Colada	5 mins	Serves 1
<ul><li>6 ounces orange juice</li><li>1 cup pineapple</li><li>½ cup fresh coconut milk</li><li>2 scoops Herbalogica Orange</li></ul>		
Combine all ingredients in a blender and blend well.		
✓ LOVED IT! ✓ Didn't like it		

Citrus Berry Splash		5 mins	Serves 1
<ul><li>2 scoops Herbalogica Orange</li><li>½ cup blackberries</li><li>¼ cup blueberries</li><li>½ cup strawberries</li></ul>	<ul><li>½ banana (optional)</li><li>The juice from 2 freshly squeezed oranges</li><li>1-2 cups ice cubes</li></ul>		
Combine all ingredients in a blender and blend well.			
✓ LOVED IT!	✓ Didn't like it		

Coconut chocolate Delight	5 mins	Serves 1

- 1 banana
- Milk from a Baby Thai coconut
- Meat from a Baby Thai coconut
- 2 scoops Herbalogica Chocolate

Combine all ingredients in a blender and blend well.

✓ LOVED IT!	✓ Didn't like it

Snack Shake	5 mins	Serves 1

- 1 scoop of Chocolate, Vanilla, Strawberry, or Orange Cream Herbalogica Nutritional Shake
- Ice and water to equal 8 oz.

Combine all ingredients in a blender and blend well.

✓ LOVED IT!	✓ Didn't like it

Meal Shake	5 mins	Serves 1

- 2 scoops of Chocolate, Vanilla , Strawberry or Orange Cream Herbalogica Nutritional Shake
- Ice and water to equal 10 oz.

Combine all ingredients in a blender and blend well.

✓ LOVED IT!	✓ Didn't like it

Salads

Confetti Salad	15 mins	Serves 2

- 1 cup Red Cabbage
- 2 cups Chopped Romaine Lettuce
- ½ cup tomato, diced
- ¼ of an avocado, diced
- 2 tbsp Annie's Lemon and Chive Dressing

Mix all ingredients and Savor! Mmmm. Tip – This salad is filling! Use it as a Main meal.

✓ LOVED IT!	✓ Didn't like it

Fennel and Orange Salad	15 mins	Serves 2

- 2 cups raw spinach
- 1 small fennel bulb, thinly sliced
- 1 orange, peeled and sectioned
- lemon vinaigrette

Combine all ingredients with desired amount of dressing.

✓ LOVED IT!	✓ Didn't like it

Green Salad	10 mins	Serves 1

- 2 cups mixed lettuce
- 4 thin slices of Roma tomato, cucumber or carrot
- 1 tbsp Choice of Dressing

Place lettuce and dressing in a bowl and toss. Transfer to plate. Garnish with tomato, cucumber, or carrot.

✓ LOVED IT!   ✓ Didn't like it

Greek Salad	15 mins	Serves 1

- 2 cups chopped romaine lettuce
- 1 Roma tomato, seeded and cut into chunks
- ¼ cucumber, seeded and cubed
- ¼ cup thinly sliced red onion
- ¼ red bell pepper, cut into chunks

Combine all ingredients with desired amount of dressing.

✓ LOVED IT!   ✓ Didn't like it

Lemon Herb Dressing	15 mins	Serves 1

- ½ cup extra-virgin olive oil
- ¼ cup fresh lemon juice
- 1 tsp. dill
- 1 tsp. oregano
- 1 tsp. tarragon
- 1 clove garlic crushed
- Dash of salt
- Dash of pepper

Place all ingredients in a bowl and toss.

✓ LOVED IT!   ✓ Didn't like it

Harvest Salad	15 mins	Serves 1

- 2 cups of torn red leaf lettuce
- ¼ apple, sliced
- 2 tbsp Vinaigrette
- 1 tbsp fresh raspberries

1. Place lettuce, apples and vinaigrette into a bowl and toss.
2. Transfer to a plate and sprinkle with raspberries

✓ LOVED IT!   ✓ Didn't like it

Mediterranean Salad	15 mins	Serves 2

- 4 Medium tomatoes
- 2 cucumbers
- 1 cup chopped fresh parsley
- ½ tbsp chopped basil
- ¼ cup extra-virgin olive oil
- ½ tsp Celtic salt
- Juice of 2 lemons

Combine all ingredients in bowl and toss well.

✓ LOVED IT!   ✓ Didn't like it

Nori and Avocado Salad		20 mins	Serves 2

- 1 cup Romaine lettuce, chopped
- 1 cup Spinach, chopped
- ½ cup alfalfa sprouts
- 4 Sheets of Nori
- ½ Avocado, diced

1. Mix ingredients in a medium salad bowl. Set aside.
2. Place a nori sheet in a frying pan on medium heat. Turn the nori from side to side until it goes from black to bright green. Repeat with other sheets of nori.
3. Cut nori into bite size pieces and add to salad. Toss well and add avocado. Drizzle "Energy Dressing" over the top. Enjoy!

*Substitute ½ cup sliced cucumber for the avocadoes for a lighter, equally delicious salad!

✓ LOVED IT!   ✓ Didn't like it

Spring Garden Salad		30 mins	Serves 4

Salad

- 4 cups chopped Iceberg or Salad Bowl lettuce
- 4 cups chopped Butter lettuce
- ½ cup chopped tomato
- ½ cup black olive
- ½ alfalfa sprouts
- ½ sunflower sprouts
- 1 cup thin broccoli florets, steamed
- 1 cup small cauliflower florets, steamed
- 1 cup cubed zucchini, sautéed
- 1 cup snow peas, blanched and halved
- 1 cup petit peas, steamed

Dressing

- 5 tbsps extra-virgin olive oil
- 2 ½ tbsps lemon juice
- 2 tbsps dairy-free mayonnaise or Almonnaise
- ½ tsp Dijon-style mustard
- Dash of Worcestershire sauce
- 2 tbsps water
- 1 tsp minced onion

1. Place lettuce in large bowl

2. Measure dressing ingredients into hand blender container and blend until creamy

3. Add tomato, olives, and sprouts to lettuce. Toss in cooked vegetables. Add dressing and toss well.

✓ LOVED IT!   ✓ Didn't like it

Dressings

Energy Dressing	5 mins	Serves 2

- 1 clove garlic, minced
- 3 tbsps Olive Oil
- 1 tbsp lemon juice
- ¼ tsp sea salt

Place all ingredients in bowl and let marinate for 10-15 minutes.

✓ LOVED IT!   ✓ Didn't like it

Italian Marinade or Dressing	15 mins	Serves 4-6

- ½ cups fresh lemon juice
- ¼ cups water
- 1/3 cups olive oil
- 1-2 cloves garlic, peeled and minced
- ¼ tsp sea salt, optional
- 1 tbsp each coarsely chopped oregano and basil

Refrigerate in jar 2-4 hours before using. Shake well before using.

✓ LOVED IT!   ✓ Didn't like it

Garlic Olive Oil Dressing	15 mins	Serves 2

- 2 cloves of garlic
- 1/8 tsp sea salt
- Juice from half of a freshly squeezed lemon
- 1/3 cup flax oil

Mash garlic cloves with Salt. Squeeze lemon juice into the mixture. Taste…if needed; add more salt, garlic, or juice. Add flax oil. Mix all ingredients together and pour over salad.

✓ LOVED IT!   ✓ Didn't like it

Dr. Julie-Ann Holland's Candida Friendly Dressing	15 mins	Serves 6-8

- ½ cup Lemon Juice
- 1 ½ cups Olive Oil
- 2 tbsp Minced Ginger
- 1/3 cup Minced Garlic

Blend all ingredients until creamy. Keeps for up to five days in refrigerator.

✓ LOVED IT!   ✓ Didn't like it

CONDIMENTS/DIPS/SPREADS/MARINADES

APPETIZERS

Chunky Guacamole		10 mins	Serves 4-6

- 1 medium avocado, peeled, pitted, and grated
- 2 tbsp fresh squeezed lemon juice
- 1 large tomato, chopped
- 2-4 green onions, chopped
- ½ tsp garlic
- Fresh pepper and sea salt to taste

Mash avocado with a fork. Chop the tomato.   Add all ingredients and mix well.

✓ LOVED IT!   ✓ Didn't like it

Classic Guacamole		10 mins	Serves 8-10

- 2 ripe avocados
- ¼ tsp garlic powder
- 1 tbsp fresh lemon juice
- ½ tsp fresh oregano
- ¼ tsp ground cumin
- Fresh pepper and sea salt to taste

Throw ingredients in a food processor. Chill, if desired, before serving.

✓ LOVED IT!   ✓ Didn't like it

Fresh Tomato Salsa		15 mins	Serves 2-3

- 3 large Roma tomatoes, peeled
- 1 tbsp crushed jalapeno peppers
- 4 green onions, chopped
- 2 tbsps fresh lime juice
- Pinch of finely chopped red chili peppers

1. Chop the tomatoes into small pieces.
2. Combine tomatoes with remaining ingredients in a medium sized bowl and stir.
3. Wrap tightly and refrigerate for one day before serving or leave covered at room temperature to allow flavors to blend. May be stored in fridge for up to 2 days.

✓ LOVED IT!   ✓ Didn't like it

CONDIMENTS

Homemade Tomato Sauce		25 mins	Serves 2-3

- 2 leaves fresh basil
- Small handful loosely packed parsley leaves (about _ oz)
- 1 small onion (about 2 ounces) – peeled and cut into 8 pieces
- 1 tbsp olive oil
- 3 medium ripe tomatoes (about 18 ounces total) cored and quartered
- dash of salt
- dash freshly ground black pepper

1. Process the fresh basil and parsley until finely chopped.
2. Add the onion and chop.
3. Transfer into saucepan with the oil and cook, stirring, for 2 minutes.
4. Process the tomatoes until coarsely chopped and add to saucepan.
5. Bring to a boil; reduce heat and cook, partially covered, for 20 minutes, stirring occasionally.
6. Process the mixture all together.
7. Strain the sauce. Add salt, pepper and cook uncovered for 10 minutes more or until thick.

✓ LOVED IT!   ✓ Didn't like it

Salsa		10 mins	Serves 2

- 2 tomato, chopped
- ½ red onion, chopped
- 1 jalapeno pepper, seeds removed & chopped
- cilantro, chopped
- parsley, chopped
- juice of ½ a lime
- sea salt & pepper

Combine all ingredients and mix together. For best results let refrigerate for 1 hour before Serving.

✓ LOVED IT!   ✓ Didn't like it

SOUPS

American Vegetable Soup		1 hr 10mins	Serves 6

- 1 tbsp extra virgin olive oil
- 2 cups sliced leeks
- 1 sliced medium red onion
- 2 carrots, halved and cut 1/8 in rounds
- 1 medium green cabbage, chopped (8 cups)
- 1 tsp fresh thyme
- 7 cups boiling water
- 1 tbsp low sodium organic chicken broth
- 3 tbsp lemon juice
- 2 peeled and chopped medium tomatoes
- Freshly ground pepper
- ½ cup celery
- ½ cup green beans
- ½ cup peas

1. Heat oil, garlic, onion, and thyme and sauté until onion begins to soften (about 2 minutes)
2. Add carrots, celery, green beans, peas, and cabbage. Sauté and stir for 2 minutes.
3. Add water and bring to a boil. Stir in broth and tomato paste. Cover and bring to boil. Simmer for 35 to 40 minutes.

✓ LOVED IT!   ✓ Didn't like it

Creamy Celery Soup	30 min	Serves 4-5

- 1 medium onion
- 1 medium celery stalk
- 1 medium garlic clove
- 1 tbsp olive oil
- 4 cups chopped vegetables, in ½ to 1 inch pieces
- 5 cups low-sodium, organic vegetable broth
- Freshly ground pepper

1. Boil water
2. Chop onion and celery. Slice garlic into thin strips.
3. Heat oil, onion, garlic, and celery in a separate pot. Cook and stir for 1 minute on medium heat. Add vegetables and continue to cook for 1 minute.
4. Add boiling broth and bring back to a boil. Stir and reduce heat to medium. Cover and cook for 8-10 minutes. Simmer until vegetables are tender.
5. Pour soup into a bowl to cool.
6. Place ¾ of soup in blender and liquefy to a cream. Pour into original soup pot. Place remaining one-quarter of unblended soup in blender. Pulse-blend for 2 to 3 seconds, allowing mixture to remain lumpy and textured. Pour it into creamed portion in the original soup pot.
7. Place soup over medium heat. Gently reheat soup, taking care not to let it boil and stirring frequently. Add pepper to taste.

✓ LOVED IT!   ✓ Didn't like it

Ginger Soup	10 min	Serves 3-4

- 6 cups of water
- 2 cups broccoli
- 1 cup tofu cubes, in ½ inch pieces
- 1 cup snow peas
- 1 cup coarsely chopped watercress
- 1 (1/2-inch) slice fresh ginger, pressed in garlic press (1 tsp)

1. Boil broth. Add broccoli. Simmer for 2 minutes. Add snow peas, watercress, and ginger.
2. Stir well and simmer for another 2 minutes.
3. Remove from heat

✓ LOVED IT!   ✓ Didn't like it

Happy Vegetable Soup	15 min	Serves 3-4

- 1 small onion
- 2 green onions
- 2 celery stalks
- 2 carrots
- 1 zucchini
- 1 pressed garlic clove
- 2 green chard leaves
- 2 cups broccoli
- 1 tbsp extra virgin olive oil
- 6 cups low-sodium, organic vegetable broth
- ½ cup minced fresh parsley

1. Cut vegetables (except chard and broccoli) into ½ inch pieces.
2. Coarsely chop chard and cut broccoli into thin florets.
3. Sauté onion, green onion, celery, carrots, zucchini, and garlic in oil. Add hot broth then boil. Simmer for 5 minutes (covered)
4. Stir in parsley. Remove pot from heat and cover for two minutes

✓ LOVED IT!   ✓ Didn't like it

Vegetable Garden Soup	20 min	Serves 8

- 6 cups low-sodium, organic vegetable broth
- ½ tsp extra virgin olive oil
- 2 carrots, peeled and diced
- 1 large onion, diced
- 1 cup of chopped broccoli
- 4 Cloves of garlic, minced
- 1/2 cabbage, chopped
- 1/2 pound frozen green beans
- 2 tbsp tomato paste
- 1 tsp fresh basil
- 1 tsp fresh oregano
- 1 tsp sea salt
- 1 large zucchini, diced

1. Bring the broth to a boil
2. Put Extra-Virgin Olive Oil in Dutch oven and heat on MEDIUM HIGH.
3. Add the carrots, onion and garlic and cook for about 5 minutes.
4. Add all the remaining ingredients EXCEPT the zucchini and bring to a boil.
5. Cover, reduce the heat to MEDIUM and simmer for about 15 minutes or until the beans are tender.
6. Add the zucchini and cook until the zucchini is tender.

✓ LOVED IT!   ✓ Didn't like it

Veggie Chowder	20 mins	Serves 4

- 2 large tomatoes, peeled, cored and pureed
- 1 cup water
- 1 medium red bell pepper, diced
- 1 medium yellow onion, finely chopped
- 1 garlic clove, minced
- 1 tbsp fresh parsley, chopped
- 1 tbsp fresh sage, chopped
- 1 tbsp fresh thyme, chopped

Combine all ingredients in large pan; mix and bring to a boil. Reduce heat and simmer 10-15 minutes or until vegetables are tender.

✓ LOVED IT!   ✓ Didn't like it

Warm Vegetable Soup	15 min	Serves 3-4

- 1 small onion
- 2 green onions
- 2 celery stalks
- 2 carrots
- 1 zucchini
- 1 garlic clove, pressed
- 2 green chard leaves or kale
- 2 cups broccoli florets
- 1 tbsp extra virgin olive oil
- 6 cups low-sodium, organic vegetable broth
- ½ cup minced fresh parsley

1. Cut vegetables into ½ inch pieces except for chard and broccoli. Chop chard and broccoli into thin pieces.
2. Sauté onion, green onions, celery, carrots, zucchini, and garlic in oil in a large pot. Add water and bouillon cubes and bring to a boil. Simmer and cover for 5 minutes.
3. Add chard and broccoli to pot. Return to a boil and simmer for 5 minutes.
4. Stir in parsley. Cover and remove pot from heat and let stand for 2 minutes

✓ LOVED IT!   ✓ Didn't like it

VEGETABLE DISHES

Beet Greens and Chard	12 mins	Serves 2-4

- 1 bunch red chard
- 1 bunch beet greens
- 1 tbsp lemon juice

1. Wash and coarsely shop greens.
2. Place in a covered pan over low heat and cook for 10 minutes. Occasionally stirring.
3. Sprinkle lemon juice and toss

✓ LOVED IT!　　　　　　　✓ Didn't like it

Belgian Endive Delight	25 mins	Serves 6

- 2-3 tbsp extra virgin olive oil
- 6 Belgian endive, cut in half lengthwise
- 2 to 3 cups water
- 3 tbsp lemon juice

1. Preheat oven to 375F. Heat oil in a large skillet.
2. Add endive and brown on both sides.
3. Add water to come halfway up endive.
4. Add lemon juice, cover, and place in oven for 20 minutes (or until liquid is absorbed).

✓ LOVED IT!　　　　　　　✓ Didn't like it

Bunches of Broccoli	15 mins	Serves 1

- 1 bunch of broccoli
- 2 tbsp organic butter
- Sea salt & cayenne pepper, to taste
- 1 tsp fresh lemon juice

Steam broccoli tops until tender crisp. Drain. Melt butter in skillet over low heat. When butter begins to brown, add lemon juice, salt and pepper. Pour over hot broccoli. 3-4 servings

✓ LOVED IT!　　　　　　　✓ Didn't like it

Carrot "Stuffing"	20 mins	Serves 2-4

- 3-5 lbs. Carrots, juiced, save the pulp.
- 3 large ripe avocados
- 1 medium head celery
- 1 red onion
- 2 tomatoes

1. Mix the celery and onions in a food processor, or with the champion juicer with the blank in.
2. Add this to the carrot pulp.
3. Add diced tomatoes to the mixture.
4. Mush up 3 large ripe avocados.
5. Add and mix thoroughly.
6. Mix up and eat! (You may want to add a little bit of the carrot juice back to the mix for extra moistness and sweetness)

This can be eaten alone, added to a salad, placed on lettuce leaves, stuffed in a pepper, etc.

✓ LOVED IT!　　　　　　　✓ Didn't like it

Filled Eggplant		30 mins	Serves 4-6

- 1 medium eggplant, peeled and cubed
- 1 tsp sea salt
- 8 tsp coconut oil
- 1 medium green pepper, cored, seeded and chopped
- 2 cloves garlic, chopped

Cover eggplant in water, add the sea salt and soak for 20 minutes. Drain. Coat heated skillet in oil. Add eggplant, pepper and garlic. Cover and reduce heat to low. Cook until tender, 6-7 minutes.

✓ LOVED IT!   ✓ Didn't like it

French Garlic String Beans		35 min	Serves 4-6

- 2 tbsp extra virgin olive oil
- 1 tsp garlic, minced
- 4 cups fresh string beans, julienned
- ½ tsp dried thyme
- ½ tsp sea salt
- 2 cups water
- 3 tbsp low-sodium organic chicken broth
- Squeeze of fresh lemon juice

1. Heat oil in a large saucepan.
2. Add garlic and beans and sauté on high to sear beans, stirring frequently so they don't burn.
3. Add thyme, salt and pepper to taste.
4. Add water and chicken broth.
5. Bring to a boil, cover tightly, reduce heat to medium-low, and simmer for 20-30 minutes.
6. Squeeze lemon juice on top and toss well.

✓ LOVED IT!   ✓ Didn't like it

Garlic Green Beans		15 mins	Serves 2-3

- 2 cups fresh green beans
- ¼ cup minced onion
- 1 Clove Garlic
- 1 tsp extra virgin olive oil

1. Combine olive oil and garlic in saucepan over medium heat
2. Combine all ingredients in saucepan sauté over med heat until green beans are tender.

✓ LOVED IT!   ✓ Didn't like it

Grilled Asparagus		7-10 mins	Serves 3-4

- 2 tbsp extra virgin olive oil
- ½ tsp pressed garlic
- 1 pound thin asparagus, trimmed

1. Preheat oven to broil or heat grill to medium.
2. Combine oil and garlic in a small bowl
3. Place asparagus on grill or broiler rack and brush with garlic flavored oil. Grill for 4 to 5 minutes. Brush and turn occasionally.
4. Asparagus is ready and outer layer is crisp

✓ LOVED IT!   ✓ Didn't like it

Heavenly Marinated Vegetable		25 mins	Serves 4-6

- ¼ cup olive oil
- 2 cups of any combination of:
- Broccoli florets
- Green or red cabbage, shredded
- Cauliflower florets
- Onion, sliced
- Any color bell pepper, cored, seeded, and cut into strips
- Tomato wedges
- 3 cloves garlic, chopped
- Sea salt to taste
- 2 tbsps chopped fresh parley
- ¼ cup freshly squeezed lemon juice

1. Heat the oil in a large skillet over low heat.
2. Add the vegetables and garlic and sea salt.
3. Stirring often until vegetables are tender-crisp.
4. Stir in parsley. Cook 1-2 minutes more.
5. Squeeze lemon juice over vegetables before serving

✓ LOVED IT!   ✓ Didn't like it

Italian Green Beans		10 mins	Serves 4-6

- Sea Salt
- 1 pound tender young green beans
- 2 tsps lemon juice
- 2 tbsp extra virgin olive oil

1. Boil water in a large pot. Trim ends off beans and cut them in half.
2. Add pinch of ground rock salt to water. Add beans. Boil for 3 minutes until bright green and tender. Drain and place in ice water. Drain and pat dry.
3. Place green beans in a bowl. Sprinkle lemon juice and toss. Add olive oil and toss again. Serve chilled or at room temperate

✓ LOVED IT!   ✓ Didn't like it

Italian Zucchini		25 mins	Serves 4

- 2 large zucchini
- 1 tsp minced garlic
- 2 tbsp fresh basil
- 2 tsp fresh oregano
- 1 tsp paprika
- Freshly ground pepper

1. Cut zucchini into thin 1/8 inch strips lengthwise.
2. Combine garlic with olive oil in small bowl and add half of mixture to a large skillet with half the zucchini.
3. Season with herbs and paprika and sauté over medium heat.
4. Rotate with tongs until zucchini is bright green. Remove from skillet.
5. Repeat process with remaining ingredients. Transfer zucchini to dish and season with pepper

✓ LOVED IT!   ✓ Didn't like it

Layered Zucchini		15 mins	Serves 4

- 1 lb. zucchini, cut into ½" slices
- 1 lb. tomatoes, peeled and diced
- 1 tsp oregano
- 1 tsp minced onion
- ½ tsp sea salt
- ½ tsp garlic powder
- ¼ tsp cayenne pepper

Combine all in saucepan. Simmer until zucchini is tender

✓ LOVED IT!   ✓ Didn't like it

Lettuce Wraps	20 mins	Serves 6-8

- 2 very ripe avocados
- 3 tomatoes, diced
- ½ jalapeno pepper, diced
- 3 cloves fresh garlic, minced
- 2 tsp lime juice
- 6-8 large romaine lettuce leaves

1. In a medium bowl mash the avocado.
2. Add remaining ingredients and stir until well mixed.
3. Spread 2-3 tbsps onto lettuce leaves and wrap

✓ LOVED IT!   ✓ Didn't like it

Lemon Broccoli	10 mins	Serves 2

- 1 head of broccoli
- 1 tbsp lemon juice, fresh squeezed
- ¼ tsp lemon zest
- Salt & pepper

1. Cook broccoli in microwave according to package instructions.
2. Combine lemon juice and zest.
3. Pour over heated broccoli.

✓ LOVED IT!   ✓ Didn't like it

Marinated Tomatoes	20 mins	Serves 2

- 1 tomato, thinly sliced
- 3-4 red onion slices
- ½ tsp fresh basil
- ¼ tsp fresh tarragon
- ¼ tsp fresh oregano
- 2 tbsps red wine vinegar
- salt & pepper

1. Place tomato and onion slices in a shallow dish, slightly overlapping each other.
2. Combine remaining ingredients in a separate bowl and pour over vegetables.
3. For best flavor results refrigerate for
   several hours

✓ LOVED IT!   ✓ Didn't like it

Melted Tomato & Zucchini Wraps	20 mins	Serves 2

- 1 tbsp extra virgin olive oil
- ½ cup thinly sliced zucchini rounds
- ½ large tomato, chopped
- ½ medium yellow onion, finely chopped
- Garlic powder, to taste
- Fresh Basil, to taste
- 2 Iceberg Lettuce Leafs

1. Preheat oven to 350 degrees F.
2. Heat oil in skillet.
3. Add vegetables and seasonings; sauté until tender.
4. Spoon vegetables on cakes; cover dish with foil. Bake 10 minutes. Let cool and place in lettuce leafs

✓ LOVED IT!   ✓ Didn't like it

Mock "Mashed Potatoes"	10 mins	Serves 2-3

- 1 Head of Fresh Cauliflower
- 1 tbsp minced dried onion
- 1/8 tsp black pepper
- 1 tbsp low-sodium organic chicken broth

1. Steam Cauliflower until tender.
2. Combine all ingredients in saucepan and cook on medium heat for 5-7 minutes, stirring frequently.
3. Remove from heat and mash with potato masher for chunkier texture or puree in a food processor for smoother texture

✓ LOVED IT!   ✓ Didn't like it

Parsley and Parsnips	18 mins	Serves 4-6

- 8 medium parsnips, peeled, trimmed and quartered lengthwise
- 2 tbsp extra virgin olive oil
- ¼ cup minced fresh parsley

1. Place parsnips in a skillet with water (enough to cover). Boil then simmer covered for 5 minutes or until tender. Drain.
2. Add olive oil, parsley, and parsnips. Heat and toss

✓ LOVED IT!   ✓ Didn't like it

Sautéed Brussels	20 mins	Serves 2

- 5-6 Brussels sprouts
- 1 cucumber
- 1 orange pepper
- 1/8 cup extra virgin olive oil

Lightly steam Brussels sprouts. Slice cucumber and pepper. Combine sprouts, spinach, pepper and oil. Toss. Add salt/spices to taste.

✓ LOVED IT!   ✓ Didn't like it

Sautéed Asparagus	20 mins	Serves 4

- ½ pound asparagus, cut diagonally
- 4 cups of water
- 1 tbsp coconut oil
- Grated fresh gingerroot, to taste
- 1 garlic clove, minced
- ½ tsp sea salt, optional

1. Cover asparagus with water in pan. Bring to boil, reduce heat and cook 5 minutes. Drain.
2. Heat oil in large skillet. Add seasonings and asparagus. Sauté, stirring often, until tender.

✓ LOVED IT!   ✓ Didn't like it

Sautéed Spinach	10 mins	Serves 3-4

- 2 tbsp extra virgin olive oil
- ¼ cup sliced onion
- 1 – 10 oz package fresh spinach, rinsed and torn
- 1 clove garlic, sliced
- Sea salt, to taste

Coat skillet with oil and heat to low heat. Add spinach and garlic, stirring often until spinach is wilted. Season with salt.

✓ LOVED IT!   ✓ Didn't like it

Spicy Taco Crunch Wraps		10 mins	Serves 2

- 1 ripe avocados
- ½ large onion
- ¼ cup fresh lemon juice
- 1/8 c fresh parsley, chopped
- 1 ½ tsp sea salt
- Romaine or leaf lettuce

1. Cut the avocado into chunks, and pour lemon juice over it.
2. Chop onion in a food processor, and then add the rest of the ingredients and process until smooth.
3. Spoon into a lettuce leaf and wrap! This tastes like a taco!

✓ LOVED IT!	✓ Didn't like it

Steamed Cabbage		15 mins	Serves 2

- ½ head of Cabbage, chopped
- juice of ½ lemon
- ½ tsp dry mustard
- salt & pepper

Steam cabbage for 5-10 minutes, until slightly tender. Combine mustard and lemon juice. Pour mixture over warm cabbage and season with salt and pepper

✓ LOVED IT!	✓ Didn't like it

Stir Fry		20 mins	Serves 2-3

- 4 tsp Coconut oil
- 1 pound vegetables: Broccoli, cauliflower, onions, and green pepper
- 1 tbsp minced garlic
- 1 tsp fresh lemon juice

1. Heat oil in skillet over low heat.
2. Add garlic and veggies. Cook until tender-crisp.
3. Stir in lemon juice. 4 servings

✓ LOVED IT!	✓ Didn't like it

Stir Fried Cucumbers		15 mins	Serves 1

- 3 medium cucumbers
- 2 tbsp coconut oil
- 2 cloves garlic, slice

Peel and halve cucumbers lengthwise; remove seeds. Cut into 1" chunks. In skillet heat oil on low heat. Add cucumbers and garlic

✓ LOVED IT!	✓ Didn't like it

Stir Fried Cabbage		15 mins	Serves 4

- 1 small head cabbage, coarsely shredded
- 3 tbsp coconut oil
- Sea salt to taste

Heat oil in skillet on low. Add cabbage, stirring until coated. Cook until tender-crisp. Season with salt, if desired

✓ LOVED IT!	✓ Didn't like it

Tasty Marinated Vegetables	25 mins	Serves 6

- 2/3 cup fresh lemon juice
- 2-4 garlic cloves, chopped
- 2 tsp total fresh parsley, basil, dill, celery seed or fennel
- 1 cup extra virgin olive oil
- 4 pounds vegetables and/or sprouts
- ½ tsp sea salt, optional

1. Combine lemon juice, garlic and herbs. Simmer 5 minutes. Cover and set aside.
2. Add oil when cooled to lukewarm.
3. Cut vegetables in 1-2" pieces.
4. Steam vegetables such as cauliflower, broccoli or green beans first.
5. Toss all ingredients together.
6. Add green onion if desired.
7. Pour marinade over and toss.
8. Marinate overnight in refrigerator

✓ LOVED IT!   ✓ Didn't like it

Tomato Cups	15 mins	Serves 6

- 6 medium tomatoes
- ½ small cucumber
- 2 sticks of celery
- ½ cup fresh parsley
- 1 tbsp fresh mint
- 1 clove fresh garlic
- 2 tsps kelp
- 1 tbsp lemon juice
- 1 tbsp extra virgin olive oil
- Sea salt to taste

Cut tomatoes in half, scoop out the center and add tomato guts to the other ingredients. Finely chop all the ingredients, mix well and fill tomato halves

✓ LOVED IT!   ✓ Didn't like it

Vegetable Delight	10 mins	Serves 5

- 1 cup Swiss chard
- 1 cup cauliflower
- 1 cup broccoli
- 1 cup carrots
- 1 cup onions
- 4 tsps coconut oil

1. Steam Swiss chard, cauliflower, broccoli, carrots, and onions until tender-crisp (about 3 minutes).
2. Coat skillet with oil and add vegetables. Stir fry about 3 minutes.

✓ LOVED IT!   ✓ Didn't like it

Vegetable Stuffed Green Peppers	15 mins	Serves 2

- 1 Green Pepper
- 1-2 cups of cooked vegetables

1. Cut peppers in half, remove stem and seeds.
2. In saucepan over low heat in 1 inch water cook covered until tender.
3. Drain. Fill with drained combination of cooked vegetables of your choice

✓ LOVED IT!   ✓ Didn't like it

Veggie Kabobs		30 mins	Serves 6

Marinade

- 2 tbsps coconut oil
- 3 tbsps chopped fresh rosemary
- 2 garlic cloves, peeled and crushed
- Juice of 2 lemons

Kabob

- 1 red bell pepper, seeded and cut into 2" cubes
- 1 yellow pepper, seeded and cut into 2" cubes
- 1 green pepper, seeded and cut into 2" cubes
- 1 onion cut into 2" cubes
- 24 cherry or grape tomatoes
- 12 wooden skewers

1. Mix marinade. Add vegetables, turning to coat all sides.
2. Refrigerate 1 hour.
3. Divide the vegetables among 12 skewers and grill for 3 – 5 minutes, brushing on extra marinade and turning

✓ LOVED IT!   ✓ Didn't like it

Wonderful Steamed Artichokes		50 mins	Serves 4

- 4 artichokes
- 1 bay leaf
- Several slices of lemon

- 6 peppercorns
- 1 garlic clove

1. Wash artichokes.
2. Put water in a steaming pot. Add bay leaf, lemon slices, peppercorns, and garlic. Put a steamer tray over the water and bring to a boil.
3. Place artichokes on a tray with their leaves down and stems up.
4. Steam for 30 to 45 minutes. When an inner leaf is easily removed you know they are done.
5. Cut off the stem of the artichoke. Cut in half lengthwise and remove the fuzzy chokes with a spoon.
6. Rub the cut sides with the lemon wedge.
7. Place in medium saucepan and add water. Bring to a boil. Cover and reduce the heat to low and cook until tender. (25-30 minutes)
8. In a small bowl, combine the oil, lemon juice and garlic.
9. Drain the artichoke and serve with dip on the side

✓ LOVED IT!   ✓ Didn't like it

DESSERTS

Banana Papaya Pudding	5 mins	Serves 2

- 1 banana
- 1 papaya

1. Cut papaya in half and remove seeds.
2. Remove inside meat and place meat with bananas in blender.
3. Blend till smooth

✓ LOVED IT!   ✓ Didn't like it

Banana Ice Cream	5 mins	Serves 2

- 2-3 Frozen Bananas (freeze without peel)

Blend frozen bananas in food processor until very smooth. Bananas may look gritty but keep blending till smooth.

✓ LOVED IT!   ✓ Didn't like it

Juice Pops	5 mins	Serves 6

- 4 Oranges
- 2 cups Berries

1. Blend berries and oranges until smooth.
2. Pour mixture in Popsicle holders or ice cube trays.
3. Insert Popsicle sticks and freeze in freezer.

✓ LOVED IT!   ✓ Didn't like it

DETOX MIXTURE

Detox Mixture	5 mins	Serves 1

- 1 ½ cups fresh lemon juice
- 2 quarts Distilled Water
- 1/3 cup pure maple syrup (for women)
      Or
- ½ cup pure maple syrup (for men)

✓ LOVED IT!   ✓ Didn't like it

CALORIE INDEX

Vegetables	Serving Size	Calories (Raw)
Artichokes	½ Cup	30
Alfalfa sprouts	½ Cup	28
Asparagus	1 Cup	27
Avocadoes	1	322
Bamboo shoots	1 Cup	41
Bean sprouts	1 Cup	53
Beets	1 Cup	58
Bok choy	½ Head	50
Broccoli	1 Cup	30
Brussels sprouts	1 Cup	38
Buckwheat sprouts	1 Cups	583
Cabbage, Chinese	1 Cup Shredded	9
Cabbage, Red	1 Cup Shredded	28
Carrots	1 Cup Chopped	52
Cauliflower	1 Cup	25
Celery	1 Cup Diced	19
Chard, Swiss	1 Cup	7
Chives	1 Tbsp Chopped	1
Cucumber	1 Cup	16
Eggplant	1 Cup Cubes	20
Edamame	½ Cup	100
Fennel, Bulb	1 Cup	27
Garlic	1 Clove	4
Green Beans	1 Cup	40
Green Onions	1 Cup Chopped	32
Jicama	1 Cup	46
Kohlrabi	1 Cup	36
Lima Beans	1 Cup	176
Leek	1 Cup	54
Mung Bean Sprouts	1 Cup	31
Okra	1 Cup	31
Onion	1 Cup	64
Parsley	1 Cup	22
Parsnips	½ Cup	100
Pepper, Green	1 Cup	30
Pepper, Red	1 Cup	48

	Serving Size	Raw
Pimentos	2 Tbsp	80
Radish	1 Cup	19
Rhubarb	1 Cup	26
Rutabaga	1 Cup	50
Shallots	½ Cup	60
Snap Beans (Edible Pods)	1 Cup	34
Snow Peas (Sugar Peas)	1 Cup	41
String Beans	½ Cup	30
Sprouts	1 Cup	56
Tomatillo	½ Cup	21
Turnips	1 Cup	36
Water Chestnuts	1 Cup	80
Wheat Grass	100 ml	14
Zucchini	1 Cup	20

Greens	Serving Size	Raw
Arugula	½ Cup	3
Beet Greens	1 Cup	8
Belgian endive	1	15
Bib lettuce	1 Cup	7
Boston lettuce	1 ½ Cup	15
Butter Lettuce	1 Cup	7
Cress	1 Cup	16
Collard Greens	1 Cup	11
Curly Endive	½ Cup	4
Dandelion Greens	1 Cup	25
Endive	½ Cups	4
Endigia (Red Endive)	½ Cup	4
Escarole	1 ½ Cup	15
Green Leaf	1 ½ Cup	15
Iceberg	1 Cup	8
Kale	1 Cup	34
Mesclun	1 Cup	10
Mustard Greens	1 Cup	15
Oakleaf	½ Cup	4
Radicchio	1 Cup	9
Red Leaf	1 ½ Cup	15
Romaine	½ Cup	5
Spinach	1 Cup	7
Swiss chard	1 Cup	7
Watercress	1 Cup	4

Fruit	Serving Size	Raw
Avocadoes	1	240
Apples	1 Cup	65
Apricots	1 Cup	74
Bananas	1 Cup	200
Blackberries	1 Cup	62
Blueberries	1 Cup	83
Boysenberries	1 Cup	66
Cantaloupe	1 Cup	60
Cherries	1 Cup	90
Coconut Meat	1 Cup	283
Dates	1	35
Figs	1	47
Grapefruit	1 Cup	97
Grapes	1 Cup	62
Guava	1	45
Honeydew	1 Cup	64
Kiwi	1 Cup	108
Lemon	1 Cup	61
Limes	1	20
Mango	1	130
Melons	1	60
Mulberries	1 Cup	80
Nectarines	1	70
Oranges	1 Cup	80
Papaya	½ Cup	70
Peaches	1 Cup	66
Pears	1 Cup	96
Persimmon	1	32
Pineapple	1 Cup	78
Plums	1 Cup	76
Pomegranate	1	105
Raspberries	1 Cup	64
Strawberries	1 Cup	49
Tangelos	1	60
Tangerines	1 Cup	80
Tomatoes	1	15
Watermelon	1	46

Dairy		
Organic butter	1 Tbsp	100
Oils		
Coconut Oil- (A great substitute for Butter	1 Tbsp	125
Extra-virgin olive oil	1 Tbsp	120
Flaxseed Oil- (Great for dressings. Keep refrigeration, do no heat)	1 Tbsp	130
Grape seed oil	1 Tbsp	120

SHOPPING LIST

Vegetables

Fresh or frozen only, organic if possible

Artichokes
Alfalfa sprouts
Asparagus
Avocadoes
Bean sprouts
Beets
Bok Choy
Broccoli
Brussels sprouts
Cabbage, Chinese
Cabbage, Red
Carrots
Cauliflower
Celery
Cucumber
Eggplant
Garlic
Green Beans
Green Onions
Lima Beans
Leek
Onion
Parsley
Parsnips
Pepper, Green
Pepper, Red
Snap Beans (Edible Pods)
Snow Peas (Sugar Peas)
String Beans
Sprouts
Zucchini

Greens

Arugula
Boston lettuce
Butter Lettuce
Collard Greens
Green Leaf
Iceberg
Kale
Mesclun
Radicchio
Red Leaf
Romaine
Spinach

Swiss chard
Watercress

Fruits

Avocado
Apples
Apricots
Bananas
Blackberries
Blueberries
Boysenberries
Cantaloupe
Cherries
Dates
Grapefruit
Grapes
Honeydew
Kiwi
Lemon
Limes
Mango
Melons
Nectarines
Oranges
Papaya
Peaches
Pears
Persimmon
Pineapple
Plums
Raspberries
Strawberries
Tangerines
Tomatoes
Watermelon

Oils

Coconut Oil
Flaxseed Oil
Grape seed oil
Extra Virgin Olive Oil

Dairy:

Organic Butter

Condiments

Real Sea Salt
Fresh Spices and seasonings
Fresh Basil/ oregano etc.

Beverages

Distilled water (Use on detox)
Spring Water
Purified Water
Fresh Squeezed Vegetable Juice

EXAMPLE MENU

Excluding detox days.

BREAKFAST

Bowl of sliced fruit with squeeze of lemon

Banana

OR

Morning Energizer

Sliced Pineapple

LUNCH

Garden Salad with Garlic Olive Oil Dressing

Sliced Apple

OR

Lettuce Wrap with Fresh Mango Salsa

Orange slices

DINNER

Garden Salad

Sautéed Mushrooms

OR

Spicy Taco Crunch

Tomato Cups

	Day 1	Day 2	Day 3	Day 4	Day 5	Day 6	Day 7
Breakfast	Breakfast: - Fruit - Vegetables	Breakfast: - Fruit - Vegetables	NO FOOD TODAY Make Detox Mixture	NO FOOD TODAY Make Detox Mixture	NO FOOD TODAY Make Detox Mixture	Breakfast: - Vegetable - Fruit	Breakfast: - Meal Shake
Snack	Snack: -Snack Shake	Snack: -	Snack:	Snack:	Snack:	Snack: -	Snack: -
Lunch	Lunch: - Lettuce Wraps	Lunch: - Confetti Salad	Lunch:	Lunch:	Lunch:	Lunch: - Confetti Salad	Lunch: - Melted Tomato & Zucchini Wraps
Snack	Snack: -	Snack: - Snack Shake	Snack:	Snack:	Snack:	Snack: - Snack Shake	Snack: - Snack Shake
Dinner	Dinner: - Steamed Artichokes -Any Salad	Dinner: - Sautéed Brussels -Any Salad	Dinner:	Dinner:	Dinner:	Dinner: -Steamed Artichokes -Any Salad	Dinner: - Bunches of Broccoli -Any Salad
Other	Other: - Can replace a meal with the NUTRITIONAL SHAKE	Other: - Can replace a meal with the NUTRITIONAL SHAKE	Other:	Other:	Other:	Other: - Can replace a meal with the NUTRITIONAL SHAKE	Other: -Can replace a meal with the NUTRITIONAL SHAKE

*Please note that you will still have to add your calories and adjust quantity accordingly.

	Day 8	Day 9	Day 10	Day 11	Day 12	Day 13	Day 14
Breakfast:	- Fruit - Vegetables	- Fruit - Vegetables	- Fruit - Vegetables	- Meal Shake	- Fruit - Vegetables	- Meal Shake	- Meal Shake
Snack:	- Fresh Veggies dipped in salsa	- Snack Shake	-	- Snack Shake	- Snack Shake	- Snack Shake	- Snack Shake
Lunch:	- Lettuce Wraps with Guacamole	- Confetti Salad	- Melted Tomato & Zucchini Wraps	- Confetti Salad Wraps	- Picnic Lettuce Wraps	- Lettuce Wraps with variety of fresh veggies	- Lettuce Wraps
Snack:	- Snack Shake	- Snack Shake	- Snack Shake	-	-	- Fresh Veggies dipped in mashed avocados	-
Dinner:	- Stir Fry - Any Salad	- Sautéed Brussels - Any Salad	- Veggie Chowder - Any Salad	- Stir Fry - Any Salad	- Lettuce Wraps - Any Salad	- Steamed Artichokes - Lettuce Wraps	- Spicy Taco Crunch - Lettuce Wraps
Other:	- Can replace a meal with the NUTRITIONAL SHAKE	- Can replace a meal with the NUTRITIONAL SHAKE	- Can replace a meal with the NUTRITIONAL SHAKE	- Can replace a meal with the NUTRITIONAL SHAKE	- Can replace a meal with the NUTRITIONAL SHAKE	- Can replace a meal with the NUTRITIONAL SHAKE	- Can replace a meal with the NUTRITIONAL SHAKE

*Please note that you will still have to add your calories and adjust quantity accordingly.

	Day 15	Day 16	Day 17	Day 18	Day 19	Day 20	Day 21
Breakfast:	- Fruit - Vegetables	- Fruit - Vegetables	- Fruit - Vegetables	- Fruit - Vegetables	- Meal Shake	- Fruit - Vegetables	- Meal Shake
Snack:	- Fresh Veggies dipped in mashed avocados	- Snack Shake	- Fresh Veggies dipped in salsa	- Snack Shake	- Fresh Veggies dipped in salsa	- Snack Shake	- Fresh Veggies dipped in salsa
Lunch:	- Lettuce Wraps with variety of fresh veggies Dressing	- Any Salad	- Any Salad with Fresh Tomato Salsa	- Mediterranean Salad	- Any Salad with Guacamole	- Veggie Kabobs with Italian Marinade or Dressing	- Lettuce Wraps with Any Salad
Snack:	- Snack Shake	- Fresh Veggies dipped in salsa	- Snack Shake	- Fresh Veggies dipped in mashed avocados	- Snack Shake	- Fresh Veggies dipped in salsa	- Snack Shake
Dinner:	- Vegetable Stuffed Green Peppers -Any Salad Fresh Vegetables	- Sautéed Asparagus -Any Salad	- Sautéed Spinach -Any Salad	- Veggie Kabobs -Any Salad	- Vegetable Delight -Any Salad	- Marinated Vegetables -Any Salad	- Marinated Vegetables -Any Salad
Other:	- Can replace a meal with the NUTRITIONAL SHAKE	- Can replace a meal with the NUTRITIONAL SHAKE	- Can replace a meal with the NUTRITIONAL SHAKE	- Can replace a meal with the NUTRITIONAL SHAKE	- Can replace a meal with the NUTRITIONAL SHAKE	- Can replace a meal with the NUTRITIONAL SHAKE	- Can replace a meal with the NUTRITIONAL SHAKE

*Please note that you will still have to add your calories and adjust quantity accordingly.

CHB10 –Enjoy Water – Nature's Elixir for Health

Water is critical to the treatment of any health condition, including candida. Every organ of the body requires water. During this session, you will build your desire for water and supercharge your motivation to drink all that your body needs for flushing toxins and healing every cell. Through the power of thought, you will build the habit of drinking water while regaining your taste for nature's health elixir. There are no substitutes for water, and soon you'll be that person who will not settle for less than the best for your body. Visualizing drinking enough water each day and then doing it will=have you feeling more energetic and positive than you've dreamed possible.

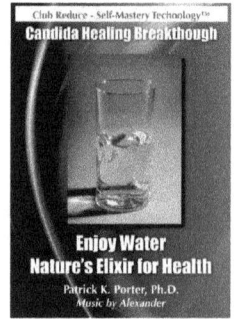

CHB11 – Unlock Your Body's Innate Healer

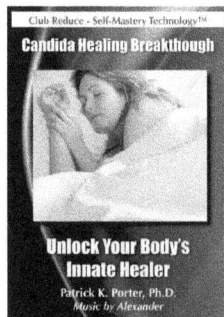

During this SMT session, Dr. Porter will help you tap into your inner healer. By following Club Reduce's core values of beautify and better the body through researched methods, this visualization will help you relax and let that power greater than yourself do the work. When you get out of the way and allow the Club Reduce program to do what it does naturally, your body's own ability to achieve optimum health will transform your experience—and isn't that better than harmful chemicals, surgery, or addictive drugs?

CHB12 – Put Your Candida-Free Lifestyle on Auto-Pilot

Dr. Porter will guide you through a timeline of change so that what you learned over the last 12 weeks will be locked into your mind and show up as new behaviors, a new attitude and positive core beliefs that will keep you candida free for life. You will experience the new energy and joy of taking back control. With this breakthrough lesson in life mastery, you will gain conscious tools to keep you on track with your health as naturally as you are breathing.

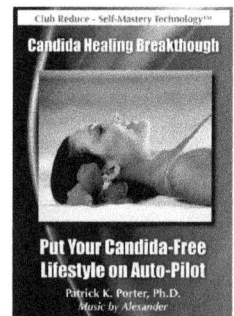

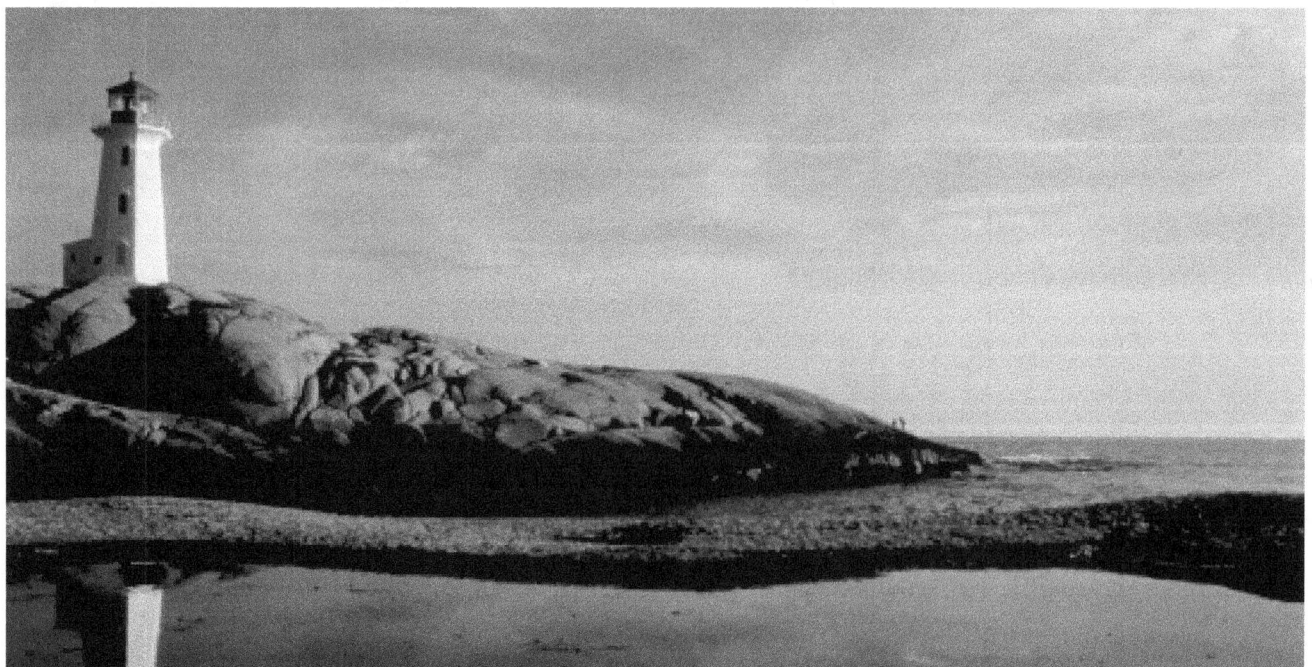

Club Reduce

Neuropathy Breakthrough Program

People with or without diabetes can develop neuropathy over time resulting in damage throughout the body. Whether you have nerve damage or have no symptoms at all, there is no better way to bring your body into balance than with this breakthrough program developed by the founder of Club Reduce, Todd Singleton, D.C. and the creator of Self-Mastery Technology (SMT), Patrick K. Porter, Ph.D.

The program is designed to work hand in hand with the nutritional protocols developed by Dr. Todd Singleton and used by Club Reduce doctors across the country for the past 20 years. If you're experiencing symptoms such as pain, tingling, numbness or loss of feeling in the hands, arms, or legs, the Neuropathy Breakthrough Program is for you.

Each SMT audio-session is designed to work with your body's intelligence and with the world-class nutritional products provided by Herbalogica to speed up the healing process. The meal plans included in this program will prevent nerve damage from occurring in every organ of the body including the digestive track. By focusing on controlling blood sugar and reducing stress, we have designed a one-of-a-kind program that will bring blood fat, blood pressure and your weight under control.

NB01 - The Power that Made the Body Can Heal the Body

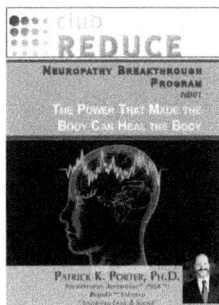

The first session from the Neuropathy Breakthrough Program is designed to adjust your thinking. Dr. Patrick Porter will be your guide in eliminating the negative thoughts that others may have instilled in you. You may have been told that there is nothing that can be done to relieve your symptoms or that you have to live with neuropathy for the rest of your life. Ridding your mind from this negativity is the first step on the road to a normal and productive life without the numbness, tingling or pain in your extremities that have troubled you in the past.

NB02 - Change Your Mind, Change the Pain and Numbness

The next step in your journey of wellness is to train your brain to trigger the most powerful pharmacy on earth – your brain. During this SMT audio-session, Dr. Patrick Porter will teach you how to tap into your brain's potential for alleviating pain when you need it most. You will learn useful techniques that you will be able to practice on your own. This session will empower you to build an optimistic outlook on life, free from the stress of neuropathy.

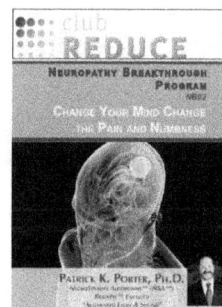

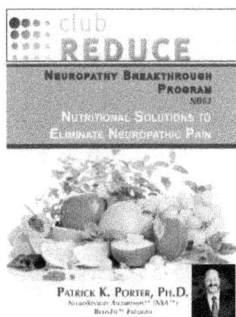

NB03 - Nutritional Solutions to Eliminate Neuropathic Pain

Based on Dr. Todd Singleton's extensive research and experience with the thousands of patients he has helped over the years, this SMT audio-session will help you create a timeline of success that includes the proven nutrition of Herbalogica as well as the in-office part of the program. In the end, all of the elements of the Neuropathy Breakthrough Program come together to help put an end to your pain.

NB04 - Balancing Blood Flow for Greater Circulation

During this SMT audio-session, you will experience a phenomenon called the relaxation response. You will have the profound realization that with relaxation comes blood flow and pain reduction. Dr. Patrick Porter will train you to respond in a healthy way to when the ravages of stress show up in your life. Sit back, relax and let go as the innate intelligence takes back control over the natural healing process of the body.

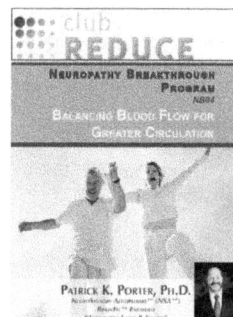

NB05 - Balancing Blood Sugar - Your Key to Being Neuropathy-Free

The Neuropathy Breakthrough Program features several components, including a comprehensive meal plan. During this SMT audio-session, you will use the power of possibility to work the program in your mind and then follow through with the physical action steps that will bring about your healing breakthrough. Dr. Patrick Porter will help you develop the mind set that you can control blood sugar one healthy meal at a time.

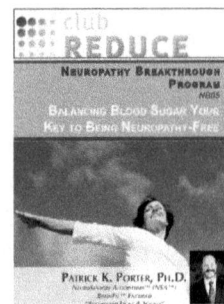

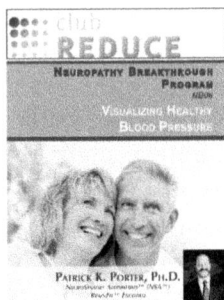

NB06 - Visualizing Healthy Blood Pressure

Research has shown that stress reduction through visualization can significantly lower blood pressure. In this SMT audio-session, Dr. Patrick Porter will teach you the skills you need to thrive without the unnecessary burden of unhealthy stress. You will also be reinforcing the healthy eating habits that will assist your body in maintaining proper blood pressure.

NB07 - Developing a Healthy Lifestyle - Exercising

During this SMT audio-session, you will begin developing a healthy lifestyle by visualizing your exercise program. Walking, running, swimming or other physical exercise will help increase blood flood in your body and speed up the healing process. This session will help you regain the physical balance and confidence you need to get started.

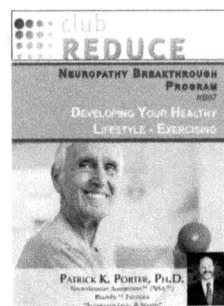

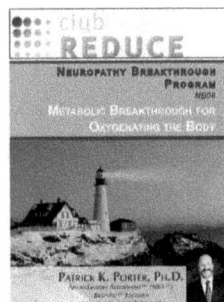

NB08 - Metabolic Breakthrough for Oxygenating the Body

During this SMT audio-session, you will reinforce the importance of bringing more oxygen into your body. Dr. Patrick Porter will guide you through deep breathing techniques. You will discover ways to exercise with oxygen that will put you firmly on the path to wellness with the help of your Club Reduce Doctor.

NB09 – Unlocking the Innate Intelligence of the Body

As your body continues to respond to the proven therapy of Club Reduce, you will see yourself returning to your natural vigor. Your energy will be replenished and you will feel young again. It is not uncommon for clients to experience a reversal of erectile dysfunction, vaginal dryness or problems with urination.

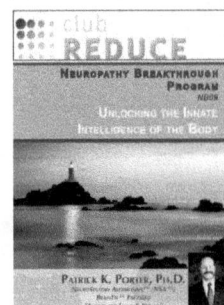

NB10 - Living Your Life Neuropathy & Drug-Free

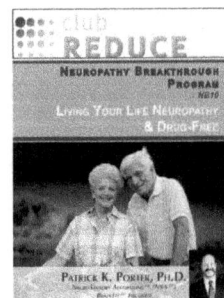

While medicine might be able to give you some relief of your symptoms, it does little or nothing to create health in the body. The Neuropathy Breakthrough Program helps you develop new healthy eating and life choices. With your newfound awareness, you will continue healing at the source by making the right food and supplementation choices, as well as by thinking like a healthy person. This is information you will want to share with your medical doctor so the two of you can work together to eliminate the need for drugs so you can live your life neuropathy-free and drug-free.

REJUVENATION PROGRAM
with Self-Mastery Technology™
Patrick K. Porter, Ph.D. & Todd Singleton, D.C.

The Club Reduce doctors spent over 20 years researching and testing methods that promote healing and weight reduction. The self-mastery program you are about to embark upon is all about getting you results. We partnered with mind-based wellness expert Patrick K. Porter, Ph.D. because our goal at Club Reduce is to help the body heal itself naturally. We know this can only happen when both your body and mind are engaged in the healing process. This program is the "missing link" to weight loss because it retrains your brain while you are retraining your body. When your body and mind are truly healthy, you will arrive at your proper weight. With the help of Dr. Porter's super-learning technology, we will educate you on how to live a new and improved lifestyle from the inside out. Our goal is to have you thinking, eating and responding to life as a naturally thin, healthy-minded person—now that's true self-mastery!

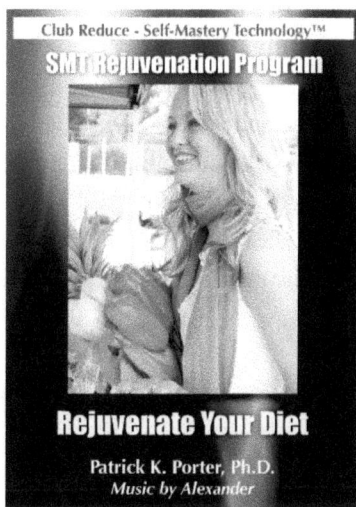

Club Reduce - Self-Mastery Technology™
SMT Rejuvenation Program
Rejuvenate Your Diet
Patrick K. Porter, Ph.D.
Music by Alexander

RVP01 – Rejuvenate Your Diet

When not detoxifying or juicing, your diet should consist mostly of green leafy vegetables. During this session, you will be guided to design a lifestyle of health and vitality in which you easily incorporate more greens into your diet. You will use the power of your imagination to create an internal timeline in which you plan meals around salads. As you learn to think like a thin person, your daily intake of fruits and vegetables will increase naturally. As your thinking changes and as your weight reduces, you will eliminate the thinking that put the weight on in the first place.

RVP02 – Detoxification— Your Key To Safe, Rapid Weight Loss

Detoxification is one of the most important factors in the promotion of good health and disease prevention. During this session, you will build the motivation to stick to your cleanse. As your body cleanses itself of toxins, mucus and other waste materials in the intestinal tract and major vital organs, improving the way they function, your positive attitude about your body and your life will improve as well, restoring vital energy to the organs and the entire body. The key here is to rid your body of toxins while cleansing your mind of any stinkin' thinkin'.

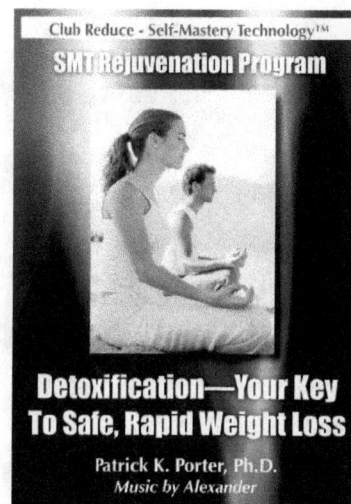

Club Reduce - Self-Mastery Technology™
SMT Rejuvenation Program
Detoxification—Your Key To Safe, Rapid Weight Loss
Patrick K. Porter, Ph.D.
Music by Alexander

RVP03 – Prepare Yourself
For A Healing Breakthrough

During detoxification and the days that follow, many people experience some of the signs of a healing crisis, which may include: headaches, skin breakouts, bowl sluggishness, diarrhea, fatigue, sweating, frequent urination, congestion, nasal discharge, or body aches. During this SMT session, you will create the mental toughness to transform the healing crisis into a health breakthrough. You will learn to relax and be patient with your body as it goes through cleansing and detoxification. You will become motivated to drink water to assist your body in its natural healing process and to use your SMT sessions to engage the amazing power of your mind.

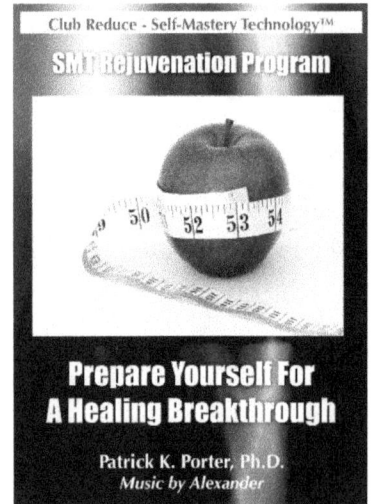

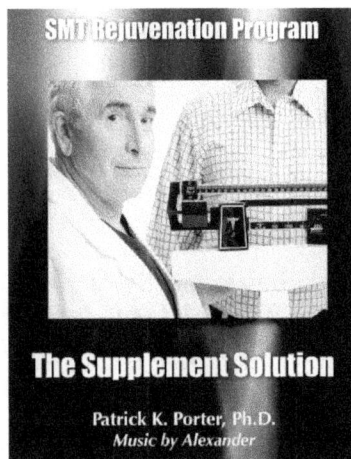

RVP04 – The Supplement Solution

Appetite happens in the mind and hunger happens in the body. Once your body gets the nutrition it needs, and your mind gets the positive stimulation it needs, you'll find it easy to eliminate emotional eating. Once you're eating to satisfy physical hunger, and not the appetite, sticking to the rejuvenation program will be a breeze. The doctors at Club Reduce searched the globe for the highest quality products and chose only those that have a direct benefit to your health. This visualization will help you get and stay motivated about using supplements for vibrant good health. While listening, you will come to understand that this will not only help you lose the weight you want, but also improve every other aspect of your life.

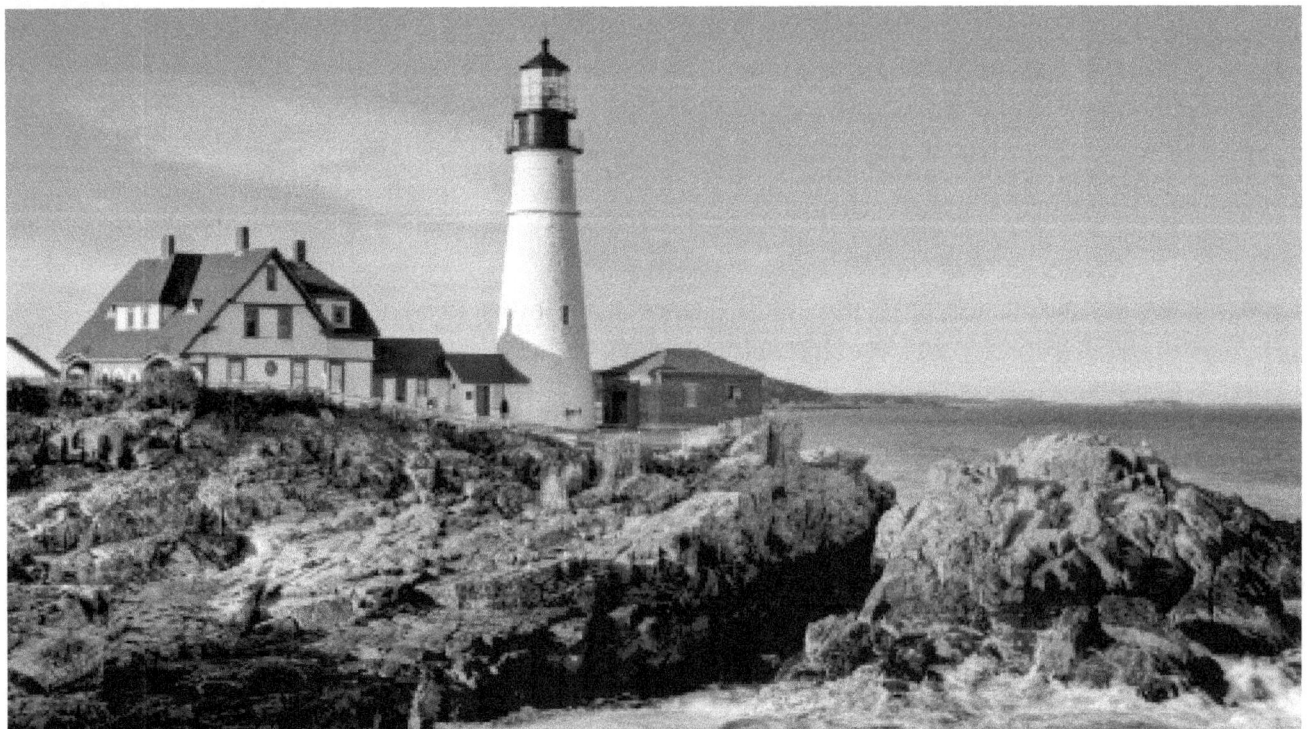

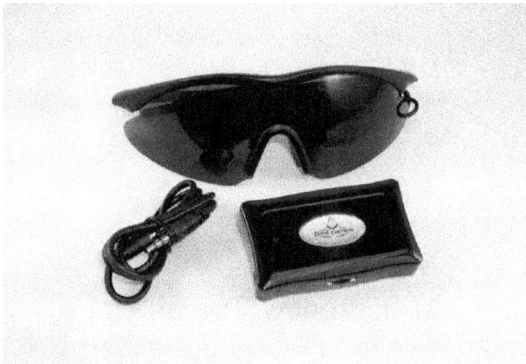

Transform Your iPod or any MP3 Player into a Portable Achievement Device

Find Out What You Can Achieve When You Dare to Relax!

ZenFrames + Your Brain = Success!

ZenFrames deliver gentle pulses of light and sound combined with guided visualization and soothing music to take you to the profound levels of relaxation known for focus, learning, achievement, and healing.

Want to lose weight? Just click on one of fifty-two titles, then relax and let your mind do the rest.

Is playing better golf your thing? Any of more than a dozen visualization sessions can easily help you master the game.

Maybe you just want a little time to get away from life's stresses. No problem. Simply choose a program from the stress-free series and enjoy a mental vacation.

A twenty-minute ZenFrames session can be equal to four hours of sleep. With hundreds of programs to choose from at ZenFrames.com, there's simply no limit to how good you can feel and what you can achieve.

If you want to get more done in less time, ZenFrames are for you!

Your ZenFrames comes with everything you need—you simply plug your ZenFrames into the earphone jack of your iPod or MP3 player and you're ready to dream big! Plus, when you register your ZenFrames, you get your own personal webpage for downloading new processes, tracking your progress and receiving updates. There's no software to install. You can take your portable achievement device with you wherever you go

Includes Six Bonus Visualization Sessions!

A $100 Value!

AM Focus
PM Dreamtime
AM Concentration
PM Release
AM Motivation
PM Success

Plus four music-only meditation sessions!

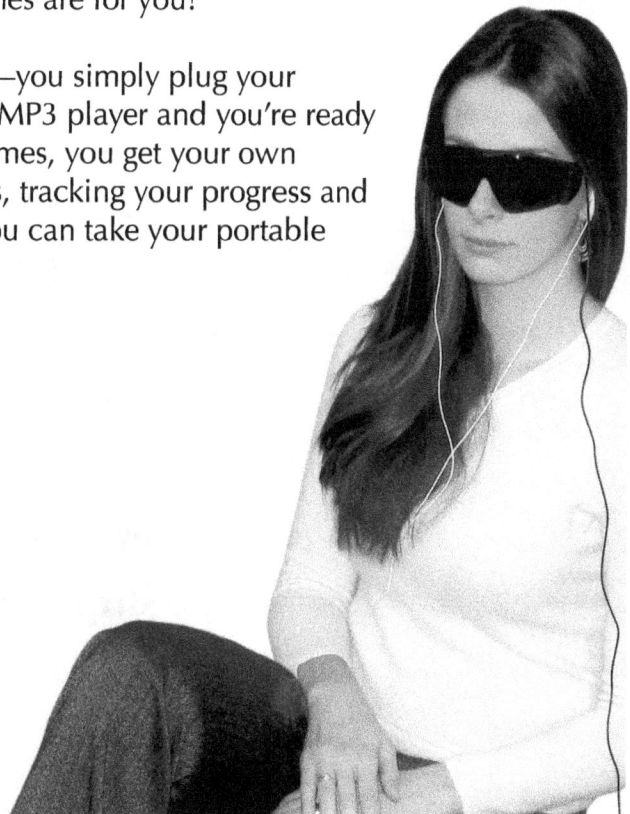

Weight Loss For Life in 10 Easy Steps

Todd Singelton, DC

Patrick K. Porter, Ph.D

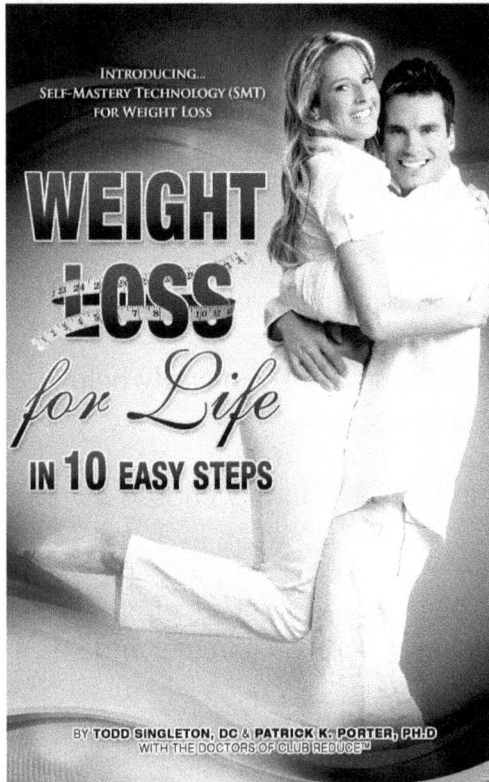

If you could lose weight on your own, you wouldn't be holding this book in your hands right now. The experts all tell you to eat fewer calories and exercise more. If only it were that easy! The truth is, most people and most so-called experts have no idea what triggers the body to gain or lose weight. Few people recognize the clues (symptoms) that are your body's warning signals that your food choices aren't working. Add the fact that almost no one understands the relationship between stress and weight, and it's no wonder we have a nation of chronic dieters who stay overweight, unhealthy and unhappy no matter how hard they try. Well, today is your day...because you have in your hands the definitive guidebook for weight loss success that lasts. Within these pages we'll teach you everything you need to know to lose weight and keep it off for life, and it couldn't be simpler when all you have to do is follow ten easy steps! Together, we'll finally make your dream a reality so you can...

- *Stop starving*

- *Be rid of cravings*

- *End emotional eating*

- *Turn off fat storage hormones*

- *Supercharge fat burning hormones*

- *Suppress your appetite naturally*

- *Clear up digestive problems*

- *Reverse the stress/weight effect*

- *Do away with habitual overeating*

- *Achieve radiant good health from the inside out!.*

Welcome to The Gift of Love Project

The Gift of Love is a poetic writing that has its own beauty … and upon further examination, it may lead one to a contemplative process, creating balance and harmony in one's everyday life. Over time, this process can also create subtle positive change in the recipient of **The Gift**.

My guidance leads me to distribute this writing to one billion people within the next two years. Hopefully, many people will be led to practice the contemplative process. If **The Gift of Love** resonates with you, please share it with others. As we gather and hold the **power of love** in our consciousness, we will dramatically reduce the level of anger, fear, and hatred on our planet today. -- Jerry DeShazo

The Gift of Love

I Agree Today
To Be The Gift of Love.

I Agree to Feel Deeply
Love for Others
Independent of Anything
They Are Expressing,
Saying, Doing, or Being.

I Agree to Allow Love
As I Know It
To Embrace My Whole Body
And Then to Just Send It
To Them Silently and Secretly.

I Agree to Feel it, Accept it, Breathe It
Into Every Cell of My Body on Each In-Breath
And On Each Out-Breath
Exhale Any Feeling Unlike Love.

I Will Repeat This Breathing Process Multiple Times
Until I Feel it Fully and Completely
Then Consciously Amplify In Me
The Feeling of Love and Project It to Others
As The Gift of Love.

This is My Secret Agreement –
No One Else Is To Know it.

For more about The Gift of Love Project and to view the videos, please visit www.TheGiftofLove.com. You will also be given access to a special 9-minute Creative Visualization that will align you with the **Power of Love** and supercharge your day. Together we will change the world one person at a time.

http://www.thegiftoflove.com/